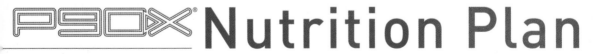

P90X Nutrition Plan

EATING FOR POWER PERFORMANCE

TABLE OF CONTENTS

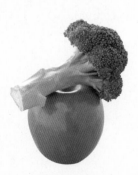

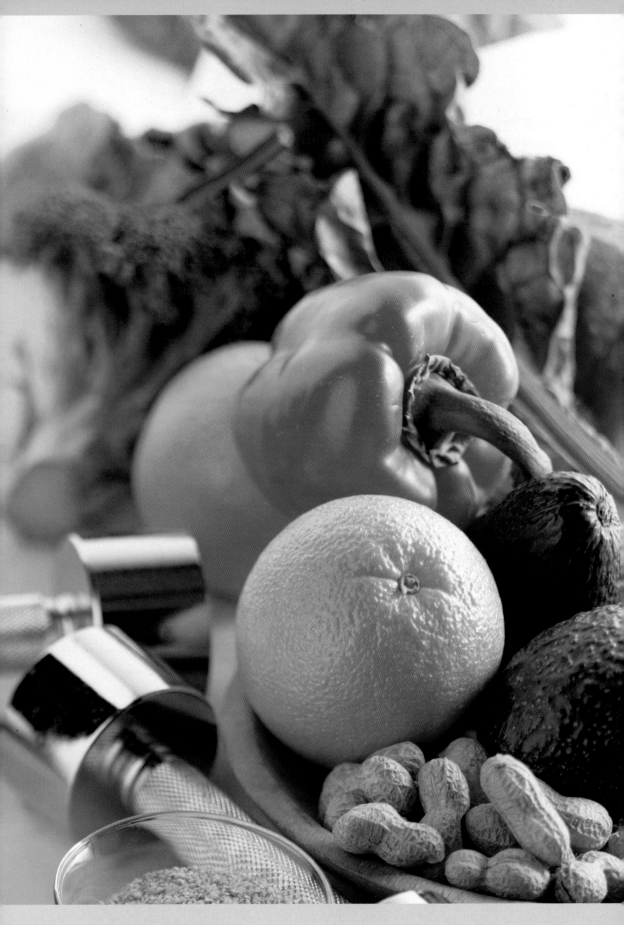

WHY THE P90X® NUTRITION PLAN LOOKS DIFFERENT FROM OTHER BEACHBODY DIET PLANS

As you may notice from the math on the following pages, P90X isn't built around a daily "calorie deficit" for weight loss like the general Beachbody plans found in Power 90®, Kathy Smith's Project:You! Type 2®, and Slim in 6®. It's important that you understand why, so you have the right training mentality with this program, with the right expectations.

Our calculations in the P90X Nutrition Plan are different from those in our other programs' diet guides and in the Diet and Support center. Running a caloric deficit during P90X is risky, and chances are it would lead to overtraining, decreased performance, or perhaps injury or illness. If someone used a 600-calorie deficit during P90X, they might see weight loss initially, but over time their performance would get worse and worse. With constant monitoring we could increase a client's caloric consumption as needed, but this isn't practical within our program structure.

To exemplify this, the number-one piece of advice we give on the Message Boards is to eat more. In the initial stages of our programs, most of our customers lose weight due to a combination of eating fewer calories, eating better calories, and increasing their workload. Over time, they stagnate—or "plateau"—at the lower caloric intake because their bodies have changed and require more calories. It's quite hard to convince them that they can eat more and not gain weight. However, it's extremely common to see our members—when on a plateau—add calories and begin seeing dramatic weight loss. We've had clients actually need to double their caloric intake before this weight loss effect of increased calories reversed. Since P90X begins at the stage where a high percentage of our clients have hit a plateau, it's important that we give them enough fuel to recover from their workouts.

Where this can go wrong is that our guidelines are ballpark and can only be ballpark. There's no way to determine exactly how individual bodies work with one document. In a lab, we could do this—obviously, a limiting factor here. With that in mind, we needed to come up with the one best solution that would fit the greatest number of people.

In my experience, Carrie Wiatt's phased diet plan was the best way to do this. I knew we would run into problems with ultrafit people attempting the initial low-carb phase. However, the point is to attempt—the best way we could within our limitations—to teach you how to determine what works for your body. The easiest way I've found is to limit carbohydrate intake until performance begins to suffer, then add them back in. Therefore, Phase 1 may last 2 months or 2 days (you need to determine this for yourself). But through the process, you'll learn what carbohydrates actually do for your body and become more sensitive to why and when you should eat them. I've used this little trick with clients for years, and especially with women, it's often the one thing that will get them off a plateau.

The bottom line is that you need blood sugar to perform your best, and this comes from eating carbohydrates. Low-carb diets can be okay for obese people in their transitioning state, but a well-fueled athletic body burns a lot of carbohydrates. This is the reason the P90X plan transitions the way it does. Real athletes do not eat "low carb" to perform and it's important to understand this.

P90X is not a fast-track weight loss solution like other programs. It's an unprecedented fitness solution designed to give you a stronger, healthier body that will become leaner and perform better over time. It's not designed for weight loss per se. It's designed to increase human performance and improve overall body composition. Trust it.

Nutrition expert Carrie Wiatt, creator of the P90X Nutrition Plan, has developed an individualized approach to healthy eating that's made her a leading lifestyle educator through her work as an author, consultant, media personality, and chef. At Diet Designs®, her Los Angeles–based nutrition company, Carrie combines fresh, upscale cuisine with low-fat preparation, portion control, and personalized counseling. After years of practice, Carrie compiled her proven techniques in her first book, *Eating by Design: The Individualized Food Personality Type Nutrition Plan*. Her second successful book, *Portion Savvy: The 30-Day Smart Plan for Eating Well*, presents a monthlong plan for controlled eating and food management. Wiatt's ability to bridge the gap between science and food circles has made her a sought-after media expert on healthy living.

As Tony Horton has been quoted as saying, your body doesn't run on exercise; it runs on the food you put in your mouth. **The goal of this guide is to help you learn what kinds of food to eat, how much to eat, and when to eat so you can lose fat, get lean, and get into incredible shape.** Be warned: If you want real results from your exercise program (AND WE MEAN *INCREDIBLE* RESULTS!), skipping this nutrition plan is NOT an option.

Establishing and maintaining the right kind of diet is just as important to your overall success as any workout. In fact, some may consider the diet the toughest exercise—but it is absolutely key to achieving your best results.

Once you incorporate the principles of the P90X Nutrition Plan into your training regimen, you will quickly begin to feel better, look better, and without a doubt perform better. Your cravings for unhealthy foods will be greatly reduced. Bye-bye, Twinkies®!

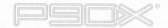

THE P90X NUTRITION PLAN HAS 3 PHASES.

This plan is designed to change right along with your 3-phase workout demands, providing the right combination of foods to satisfy your body's energy needs every step of the way.

While P90X is designed as a 90-day program, you might choose to alter your choice or timing of one or more of the plans. **You can follow any phase at any time based on your nutritional level.** These are general guidelines we're recommending.

PHASE 1
FAT SHREDDER

FAT SHREDDER
A high-protein-based diet designed to help you strengthen muscle while rapidly shedding fat from your body.

PHASE 2
ENERGY BOOSTER

ENERGY BOOSTER
A balanced mix of carbohydrates and protein with a lower amount of fat to supply additional energy for performance.

PHASE 3
ENDURANCE MAXIMIZER

ENDURANCE MAXIMIZER
An athletic diet of complex carbohydrates, lean proteins, and lower fat, with an emphasis on more carbohydrates. You'll need this combination of foods as fuel to get the most out of your final training block and truly get in the best shape of your life!

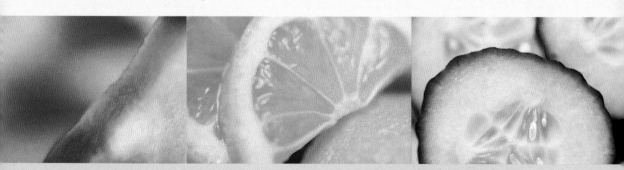

THE 3 PHASES

Like the P90X exercise program, the P90X Nutrition Guideline is divided into 3 phases, calibrated to move from fast, efficient fat loss (Phase 1) to peak energy (Phase 2) to lasting success (Phase 3). The nutritional proportions change with each plan, so it's important to follow the instructions for your current plan.

The nutritional proportions for each of the 3 plans are as follows:				
PHASE	GOAL	PROTEIN	CARBOHYDRATE	FAT
PHASE 1 FAT SHREDDER	Strengthen muscle and shed excess body fat	50%	30%	20%
PHASE 2 ENERGY BOOSTER	Maintain Phase 1 changes with additional energy for midstream performance	40%	40%	20%
PHASE 3 ENDURANCE MAXIMIZER	Support peak physical performance and satisfaction over the long term	20%	60%	20%

PHASE 1

FAT SHREDDER Those who are reasonably fit and have more body fat can use this phase more easily than someone who's very fit and doesn't have a lot of excess body fat to lose. This stage is designed to cut down your body fat percentage, and as this happens, your available energy should also decrease. Therefore, Phase 1 should only be extended if you need to drop more fat and you feel you have ample energy to push hard during your workouts. Conversely, this phase could be shortened by a week or two if your body fat is already low and you feel like you don't have the necessary energy to get the most out of your workouts.

PHASE 2

ENERGY BOOSTER This is more of a well-rounded, long-term, sensible eating plan, and there shouldn't be too much trouble once you get here. This plan can also be used as long as you like if you're feeling great, have plenty of energy, and it seems like you're making overall progress.

PHASE 3

ENDURANCE MAXIMIZER This phase should be earned. It's an athletic diet, and you'll only need it if you're pushing your body to the limit, which you should be if you keep your promise to "Bring It!®" Note that you should try Phase 3 at some point, even if you feel good in Phase 2. We've seen many people hesitate to move on to this more carb-heavy phase for fear they'll gain weight, but surprise! They found that once they did, they had more energy, worked out even harder, and had better results. This is important to keep in mind. Athletes eat more carbs, and there's a reason they do. We wouldn't put it in the plan if it weren't proven to improve results.

CUSTOMIZING THE PHASES

While P90X is designed as a 90-day program, you might choose to alter your choice or timing of one or more of the phases.

DETERMINE YOUR PHASE

- ☐ (1) FAT SHREDDER
- ☐ (2) ENERGY BOOSTER
- ☐ (3) ENDURANCE MAXIMIZER

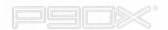

EACH PHASE HAS 3 APPROACHES.

We've developed three different approaches to ensure proper nutrition for all phases of P90X. The choice is yours as to which one will work best for you. Keep in mind that you can stick with one approach throughout the entire program, or alternate based on your lifestyle demands.

THE PORTION APPROACH

This approach is designed for those who don't have a lot of time or patience to prepare a meal that involves more than one or two steps. It's definitely better suited to those who don't like to cook or follow recipes.

THE MEAL PLAN APPROACH

By following the daily meal plans, you'll not only take the guesswork out of your daily food preparation, but you'll also enjoy a variety of delicious, healthy, and low-fat recipes that'll provide you with the proper amount of nutrition and energy to get the most out of your P90X workouts.

THE QUICK OPTION APPROACH

We all have days when it seems we can't find the time to eat, let alone cook. So we've included some quick food options that require minimal or no effort, because YOU MUST EAT TO SUCCEED WITH P90X.

DETERMINE YOUR APPROACH
☐ PORTION   ☐ MEAL PLAN   ☐ QUICK OPTION

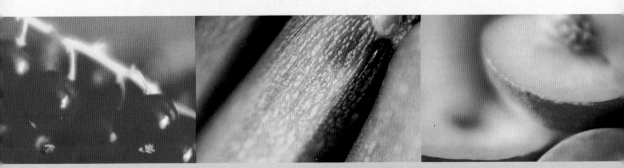

YOUR BODY FAT PERCENTAGE

Lowering your body fat and increasing lean muscle mass is essential to your overall success. It's important to track your progress by measuring and recording your body fat percentage at the end of each phase.

Use Beachbody's body fat tester to record your body fat measurements. To get the most accurate readings, follow the directions on the package. (Also record on page 16 of the P90X Fitness Guide).

	CURRENT BODY FAT %	NOTES
Start		
Day 28		
Day 56		
Day 90		

BODY FAT TARGET

As your body fat percentage changes during the next 90 days, here's where the numbers place you in terms of general targets.

	FIT RANGE	ATHLETE RANGE	ELITE ATHLETE RANGE
MEN	14–17%	10–13%	4–9%
WOMEN	21–24%	16–20%	12–15%

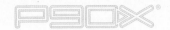

EACH APPROACH HAS **3 NUTRITION LEVELS**.

Please take a moment to determine your daily nutrition and calorie needs. The data you provide will determine how much food you need (and how much you don't need) while you go through P90X.

1

Calculate your resting metabolic rate (RMR). This is basically the number of calories you need to breathe, pump blood, grow hair, blink—be alive.

YOUR BODY WEIGHT		RMR (IN CALORIES)
	x 10 =	

2

Calculate your daily activity burn, the calories required for daily movement apart from exercise.

Keep in mind that all lifestyles aren't created equal. A construction worker will have a higher daily burn rate than

YOUR RMR		DAILY ACTIVITY BURN
	x 20% =	

a computer programmer, so this figure should be treated as a ballpark estimate. You'll probably need to do some personal adjusting to get it perfect. Don't worry; this will become more obvious than you think once you get going.

3

Add the calories required for your exercise needs, which we have calculated at 600 calories per day for the P90X program. Add it all up and you've got your energy amount.

YOUR RMR		DAILY ACTIVITY BURN		ENERGY AMOUNT
	+		+ 600 =	

4

Now use your energy amount to determine your nutrition level in the table.

Example: A 6-foot, 180-pound man

RMR = 180 (body weight in pounds) x 10 = 1,800
Daily activity burn = 1,800 (RMR) x 20% = 360
Exercise expenditure = 600
Energy amount = 1,800 + 360 + 600 = 2,760
Nutrition level = II
Round down to the bottom of your level to create a slight calorie deficit (e.g., if you're at level II, your calorie target is 2,400 calories/day).

YOUR ENERGY AMOUNT	NUTRITION LEVEL	
1,800–2,399	1,800 calories/day	LEVEL I
2,400–2,999	2,400 calories/day	LEVEL II
3,000+	3,000 calories/day	LEVEL III

YOUR NUTRITION LEVEL =

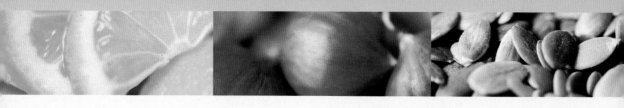

GENERAL GUIDELINES

While this plan is designed to meet each individual's nutritional needs, there are some general rules that should be applied to ensure positive results.

keeping a daily journal

Knowing what, when, and how much to eat plays a vital role in your development. In this section you'll also discover healthy ways to prepare the foods you choose to eat, and make them taste good so you'll *want* to eat them again. Following these guidelines and maintaining an eating discipline will optimize your energy level and fat-burning ability throughout your P90X workouts. Research shows that one of the most powerful ways to successfully change your eating habits is to keep a daily journal. By logging your food intake as well as your exercise, you keep yourself accountable while also creating a space to express your thoughts and feelings. You'll no longer have to remember what worked and what didn't. You can look back on your log to track your journey and fine-tune your plan according to your personal experience and needs. You'd be surprised how often bad moods are associated with bad foods.

You'll find a daily journal for each week of P90X included at the back of this book. Try to carry your current journal page with you so you can track meals as you eat them and jot down thoughts as they arise.

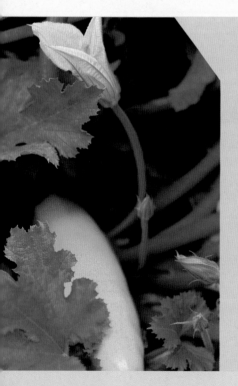

WHY DIET MATTERS

A large body of scientific evidence shows that diet and exercise work hand in hand to promote fitness and physical performance. One reason for this symbiotic relationship is the energy equation. When you expend more calories than you consume, you burn body fat (aka "stored energy") and build lean body mass—but because you need energy to exercise, every calorie you eat must be of the highest quality to get you over the hump.

As Tony says, "The better the car, the better the fuel you need to make it run as designed." We're making you into a better car, so it's time for some high-octane grub!

Another reason diet matters is metabolism. A nutrient-dense, interval-based eating program keeps your metabolic rate high to burn maximum fat, even when you're not working out. Finally, a healthy diet regulates blood sugar to balance hormonal secretions, promoting optimal fat burn and a steady fuel supply. All this works together to get you into peak condition in 90 days.

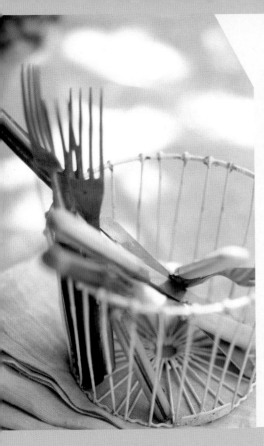

WHEN TO EAT

It's important to follow a regular eating schedule. First, it keeps your blood sugar stable instead of peaking and crashing, which can lead to overeating and a general poor feeling. Second, regular meals will speed up your metabolism by challenging it to keep processing calories, rather than storing them in a game of "feast or famine."

Success in P90X comes to those who eat early and often. You should be eating every few hours while you're awake, favoring small meals and snacks. Try to finish your last snack approximately 3 hours before you hit the sack. This'll help keep undigested carbs from being stored as fat. If you do need to break this rule, a small protein shake would be the snack of choice before bed, as it can help your recovery during sleep.

okay, let's get started.

big P90X step...   Before deciding which foods to incorporate into your selected eating plan,

TOSS THE JUNK!

Now would be a good time to get rid of all the junk food currently in your possession. Foods high in saturated and trans fats, sodium, and sugar should be the first things you throw out (e.g., cookies, pastries, candy, processed meats, potato chips, soda, high-sodium frozen foods, canned soups, etc.). You know them. You think you love them. They're the problem. Throw them away, and don't let anyone give you more. Don't be nice. Don't take a bite. Say, "Thanks, but I'm not eating that kind of stuff for 90 days." And by the way, congratulations! You're taking this program seriously, and just remember—if you think it's junk food, it probably is.

Yes, we mean it. Throw it away!

WHAT RESULTS TO EXPECT

The P90X Nutrition Plan is designed to optimize your exercise plan to build strength and lean muscle mass. This dramatic change in your physical composition means you might not see a big difference on the scale, because often you'll be trading fat for lean, strong muscle—and you'll not only see it, but you'll definitely *feel* the difference in your body. Unlike other diets that focus on the relatively meaningless measure of weight, you'll use body fat percentage and self-perceived energy to guide you to your goal. This program is for real.

THE NUMBER-ONE OBSTACLE

The number-one obstacle to success is underestimating portion size. Calories *do* count in the energy equation, and small errors can add up to big disappointments. It's very important to measure each portion accurately at every meal, the way we've outlined here. It might sound like a lot of work, but after 90 days, it'll be second nature. After 90 days, you'll know how to eat. Think of this plan as a graduate degree in eating, and you'll graduate in only 3 months.

OTHER "DON'TS" THAT CAN DERAIL YOUR DIET INCLUDE:

_ Skipping meals and eating off schedule.

_ Following fads and trends, like overemphasizing certain food groups and completely excluding others.

_ Not planning your food choices ahead.

_ Skimping on fruits and vegetables, your natural supply of antiaging nutrients.

DRINK WATER

Drinking enough water is a vital part of any conditioning program, as it aids every aspect of bodily function. You should drink at least six to eight 12-ounce glasses of water each day. The following water consumption guidelines relate specifically to your P90X workout:

P90X HYDRATION SCHEDULE

12 oz. water 2 hours prior to exercise
8 to 12 oz. water 15 to 30 minutes prior to exercise
4 to 8 oz. water every 15 minutes during exercise

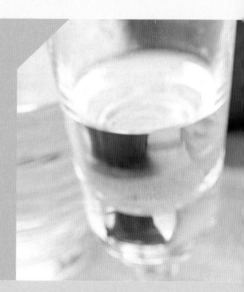

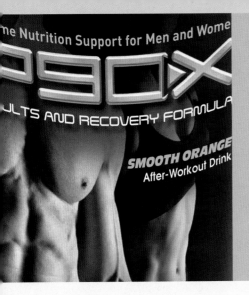

P90X® RESULTS AND RECOVERY FORMULA® AND THIS PLAN

It's best to have P90X Results and Recovery Formula after-workout drink within 1 hour of finishing your hardest workout of the day, when your glycogen stores are at their lowest. This should be the only thing you consume during this time frame. You can also split this up if you do double workouts, and have half a serving after each workout, or even a full serving after each workout if you're trying to gain mass. But keep in mind that you don't need to replenish glycogen stores if they haven't been exhausted. So if you completed one of your workouts at a lower intensity, you may want to save the Results and Recovery Formula for after your harder workout.

RECALCULATING YOUR CALORIES

Even though some pretty bright minds were tapped during the formulation of this nutrition plan, that doesn't mean it's perfect for everyone. If you feel you need to eat either more or less than you've calculated, then this really might be the case.

But first you should try eating the amount you calculated. Your body will let you know what's right over time. In the beginning, it might send you false signals, trying to get you to eat more out of habit. Given a trial period, though, your body will find its healthy balance of diet and exercise, a more accurate sense of how much you should be eating. Metabolic rates vary more than we can predict here, so there's a chance you'll need to recalculate calorie needs somewhat, either up or down.

One thing to caution you against is *undereating*. If you don't feed your body enough, your metabolism will slow down and you'll compromise your workouts. This can affect your results in ways you may not notice because you may feel okay generally, but your performance could be lagging. Don't let your energy level take a dive. The only time you should drop your caloric intake is if you're working out hard, yet still gaining fat.

You might actually need to add calories if you feel like you're running out of energy during your workouts. However, this could also result from eating too soon before you exercise. If you decide to eat more, adding as little as 200 to 300 calories per day should be enough unless your calculations are way off. You can easily up your calorie intake by adding a snack like nuts or dried fruit, substituting a meal in place of a snack, or adding a P90X Peak Performance Protein Bar or Beachbody® Whey Protein Powder shake.

"BONKING"

If you're in Phase 1, you could be "bonking" due to lack of carbohydrates in your diet. Bonking is when your body simply runs out of stored glycogen during a hard workout and can no longer push beyond its anaerobic threshold. This is very common in sports like running and cycling, but it can also happen during routine weight training, especially with a low-carb diet. In this case, adding a serving of a complex carbohydrate like brown rice, potatoes, sweet potatoes, whole-grain bread, or whole-grain pasta to any meal during the day will usually do the trick. Complex carbs are stored as liver glycogen to be used when necessary, so unlike sugars, they don't need to be consumed right before you need them in order to be effective.

LOW-FAT COOKING TECHNIQUES

Learning just a few basic skills can make you a low-fat chef with good habits you'll use for life. Cooking with liquids other than fat can trim the fat content of a dish by up to 1,000 calories. This can have a positive effect on your total health and well-being, and maybe even prevent illnesses like cancer and heart disease. And on top of all that, you can lose lots of weight.

Refer to these techniques when preparing the recipes from the Meal Plan or preparing foods from the Portion Approach.

Eliminate the fat used in traditional sautés by substituting flavorful liquids for butter, margarine, or oil. Choose chicken or vegetable stock, dry sherry, red or white wine, fruit juice, vinegar, soy sauce, or a combination of any two or more of these.

A BETTER SAUTÉ

1_ Heat 2 tablespoons of liquid in a sauté pan over medium-high heat.
2_ When the liquid begins to steam, add ingredients and stir.
3_ Continue to sauté, stirring frequently, until the liquid in the pan evaporates. Quickly add 2 more tablespoons of liquid, stirring to scrape up the glaze at the bottom of the pan.
4_ Continue to cook, adding liquid as necessary, until done.

PASTA AND NOODLES

1_ Always select pasta made without oils or eggs. All the recipes here call for dry, not fresh, pasta.
2_ Skip adding oil and salt to the cooking water; the sauce provides plenty of flavor and moisture.
3_ Cook pasta in a large pot of boiling water, adding pasta to the pot gradually so the water continues to boil.
4_ Two ounces of dry pasta yields 1 to 1-1/2 cups cooked pasta, depending on the type.

Poultry, meats, and seafood all contain natural fats and can be cooked without any additional oils. Here's how:

GRILLING, BAKING, AND POACHING

1_ Grilling is the fastest cooking method, and is best suited for thicker cuts. Begin with a preheated grill or broiler, turning meat over when the grilled side is done (fish should flake, poultry should begin to brown). Cook the other side. Depending on thickness, grill 5 to 7 minutes per side; the second side will probably take less time than the first. (Tabletop two-sided electric grills cook twice as fast.)
2_ Baking and roasting are slower cooking methods. Bake or roast most cuts at 350 degrees for 20 to 30 minutes.
3_ Poaching involves simmering slowly in liquid, like water, stock, or wine—you can flavor with herbs, onions, shallots, and/or garlic. Poaching is a gentle cooking method that works well for delicate cuts like chicken breast, fish fillets, and shellfish. In a medium to large saucepan, heat just enough liquid to cover your ingredients until it reaches a very slow simmer. Add ingredients in a single layer and cook uncovered 7 to 10 minutes, or until cooked through.

For added flavor and moisture, brush seafood, meat, or poultry with fresh citrus juice, mustard, Worcestershire sauce, soy sauce, or fresh herbs before grilling, baking, or roasting. Or use an oil-free marinade—for best flavor, marinate at least 2 hours or overnight in the refrigerator.

VEGETARIANS

If you're a vegetarian, chances are you already know this drill, but any of these P90X recipes can be prepared vegetarian-style with some creative substitutions. Keep in mind that as a vegetarian, you need to do your own calculating to get enough protein. Unlike meat dishes, most of your options contain some carbs. Here are some substitutions for meat that can help your diet stay high in protein:

_Beans/lentils/soybeans   _Nonfat yogurt
_Cottage cheese   _Seitan
_Egg substitutes   _Soy burgers
_Egg whites   _Soy cheese
_Garden burgers   _Soy yogurt
_Hemp protein   _Tempeh
_Hummus   _Tofu
_Nonfat cheese

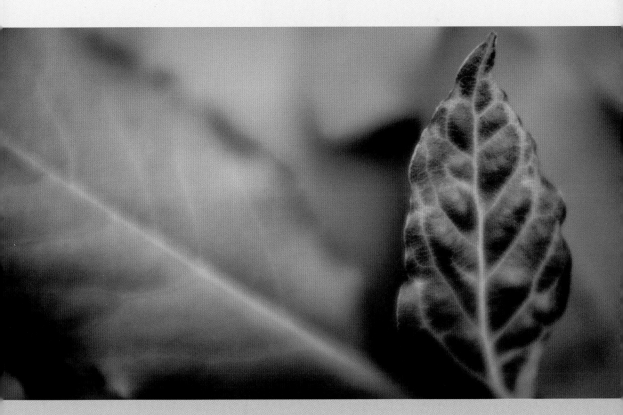

SUPPLEMENTS AND P90X

P90X RESULTS AND RECOVERY FORMULA®

There's a 60-minute window after training hard in which you need to fuel your body appropriately to maximize your results—in terms of both weight loss and performance. You'll get better results and recover faster using Results and Recovery Formula, and it tastes so great you won't believe how good it is for you. When recovering from intense workouts, this formula will provide you with the vital nutrients you need to bounce back from your workout.* And the delicious, smooth orange flavor makes it a nice post-workout reward.

A dextrose-based formula provides optimum glycogen replenishment while a high Protein Efficiency Ratio (PER) blend offers the critical building blocks for rapid muscle resynthesis. Vitamins and antioxidants help reduce muscle soreness and assist in repair and growth.*

Studies show that with proper nutrition during the first hour following exercise, you can increase your body's ability to recover by more than 100 percent. Our Results and Recovery Formula combines the proper nutrients into this state-of-the-art, great-tasting, body-shaping cocktail that's guaranteed to take your results to the next level.*

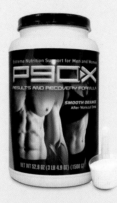

*These statements have not been evaluated by the Food and Drug Administration. These products are not intended to diagnose, treat, cure, or prevent any disease.

P90X® PEAK HEALTH FORMULA

You're doing the ultimate fitness program; it's only right that you use the ultimate supplements. P90X Peak Health Formula is the highest-quality, most complete multivitamin we've ever offered. Taken daily, each packet will ensure that your body gets the vital nutrients you need to perform at your best and get the most out of P90X.*

You may notice that the vitamin and mineral levels in Peak Health Formula go far beyond what you'll find in a conventional multivitamin. You're now exercising at a level that can seriously deplete micronutrients, so it's important to make sure you get back everything you lose—and then some.

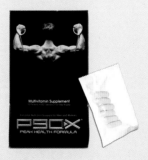

P90X® PEAK PERFORMANCE PROTEIN BARS

With four great flavors and 20 grams of protein, our bars are designed to take the edge off when you're training hard.

Yes, we spend most of this guide urging you to stay away from added sugar, but the sugar in P90X Peak Performance Protein Bars does an important job as it transports the protein to your muscles and recharges your glycogen. The fat in the bars promotes time-released delivery, because during a program like P90X, when you've incurred a ton of muscle breakdown, you're often burning glycogen even at rest trying to recover.*

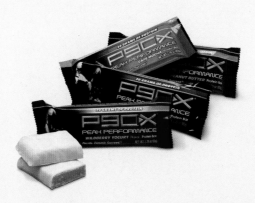

E&E ENERGY AND ENDURANCE™ PREWORKOUT FORMULA

Your P90X workouts are tough and if you don't have the energy to go full out, you won't get your best results. That's why NEW E&E Energy and Endurance™ is an essential part of your P90X workout program. It's scientifically formulated to help improve your energy, endurance, strength, and focus, so you can maximize every second of your P90X workouts!*

E&E Energy and Endurance features a proprietary blend of advanced nitric oxide boosters, amino acids, essential B vitamins, electrolytes, and natural energizers to help you power through your workouts!

E&E Energy and Endurance will help you:*
• Burn more calories and fat to get ripped faster.
• Maximize performance to build muscle faster.

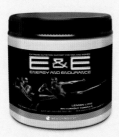

*These statements have not been evaluated by the Food and Drug Administration. These products are not intended to diagnose, treat, cure, or prevent any disease.

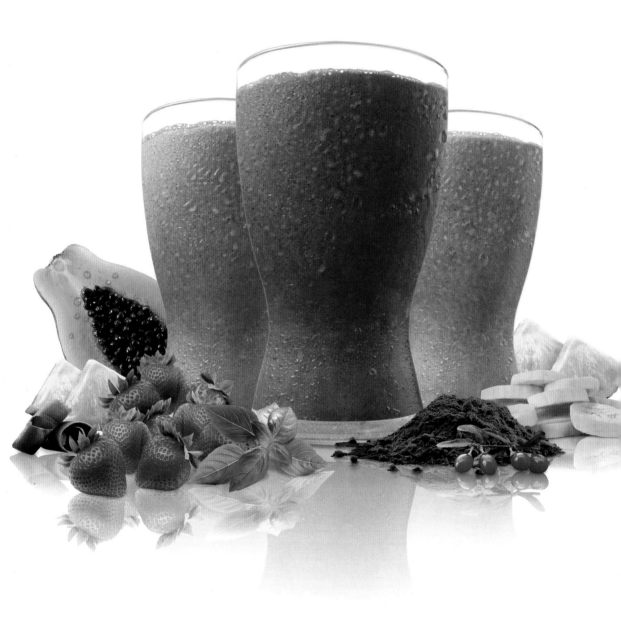

GET RIPPED EVEN FASTER.
FIRE UP YOUR ENERGY LEVELS, LOSE MORE WEIGHT, AND ACHIEVE OPTIMAL HEALTH.

Unlike any other shake out there, Shakeology® contains the most potent superfoods and essential nutrients available. Its 70-plus ingredients are derived from whole-food sources—all-natural food your body can easily absorb and utilize.

Each nutritious serving is packed with antioxidants; energy-providing carbohydrates; a full spectrum of vitamins and minerals, prebiotics and enzymes for better digestive health; and at least 15 grams of protein to keep you feeling full.* Even eating the recommended servings of fruits and vegetables every day won't give you this much nutrition.

Try it risk free for 30 days and you should notice a difference as soon as the first week. Replacing one meal a day with Shakeology can help you:
_Increase energy levels for your workout
_Reduce cravings
_Lose weight and get lean
_Improve digestion and regularity for
    optimal health

SHAKEOLOGY CONTAINS:
_Protein
_Essential Amino Acids
_Antioxidants
_Digestive Enzymes
_Prebiotics
_Vitamins
_Minerals
_Phytonutrients

How to incorporate Shakeology into P90X Nutrition Plan:
_Menu Approach: Use Shakeology for breakfast every day. Check out the recipes on pages 35 and 36.
–Portion Approach: Replace a snack or one scoop can count as ½ a Protein Portion *and* ½ a Carb Portion.

NOW AVAILABLE IN 3 DELICIOUS FLAVORS:
_Chocolate
_Greenberry
_Tropical Strawberry (vegan/dairy-free formula)

To learn more, contact your Team Beachbody Coach or visit Shakeology.com.

Follow Shakeology on: twitter

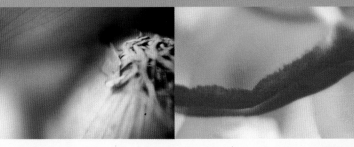

FAT SHREDDER

The Portion Approach was designed to allow you to mix and match the foods of your choice. There are NO specific meal plans or recipes for this approach. **Just select from the Portion Approach foods listed on the following pages and eat the amounts indicated for your nutrition level.** Along with identifying the right foods to buy, the list shows you which foods fall into which categories, and the appropriate portion size to equal one serving.

For example, if you're in Phase 1 and have determined that you're at nutrition level II, you'd be allotted a specific number of servings per day from each food group, as follows:

PROTEINS	7 servings	
DAIRY	3 servings	
FRUITS	1 serving	
VEGETABLES	4 servings	
FATS	1 serving	
CARBOHYDRATES	1 serving	
SNACKS	2 servings	(2 items from the single snack group or 1 item from the double snack group) PLUS a P90X Peak Performance Protein Bar and P90X Results and Recovery Formula drink
CONDIMENTS	2 servings	

Important Note on Snacks:

There are two snack groups listed in your Portion Approach foods—the single group and the double group.

If the letters **SGL** appear beside a snack serving block on your Portion Chart, you can have any 1 item from the **single snack group**. If the letters **DBL** appear inside the snack serving block, you can have any 1 item from the **double snack group** OR any 2 items from the single snack group.

Additionally, if the words **Bar** or **Drink** appear inside a snack serving block, you can have a **P90X Peak Performance Protein Bar** and **P90X Results and Recovery Formula** drink IN ADDITION TO your allotted snack servings.

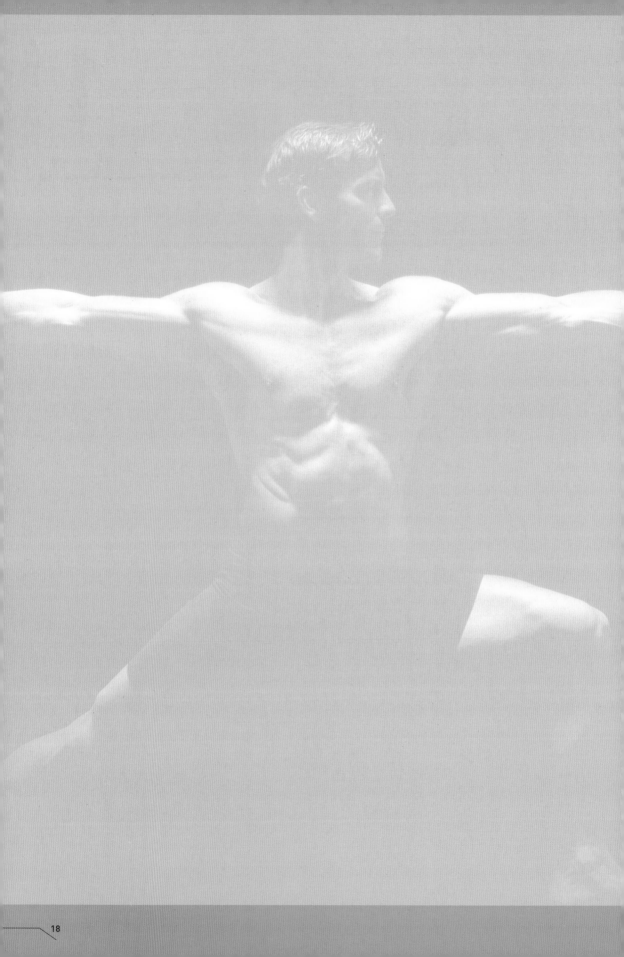

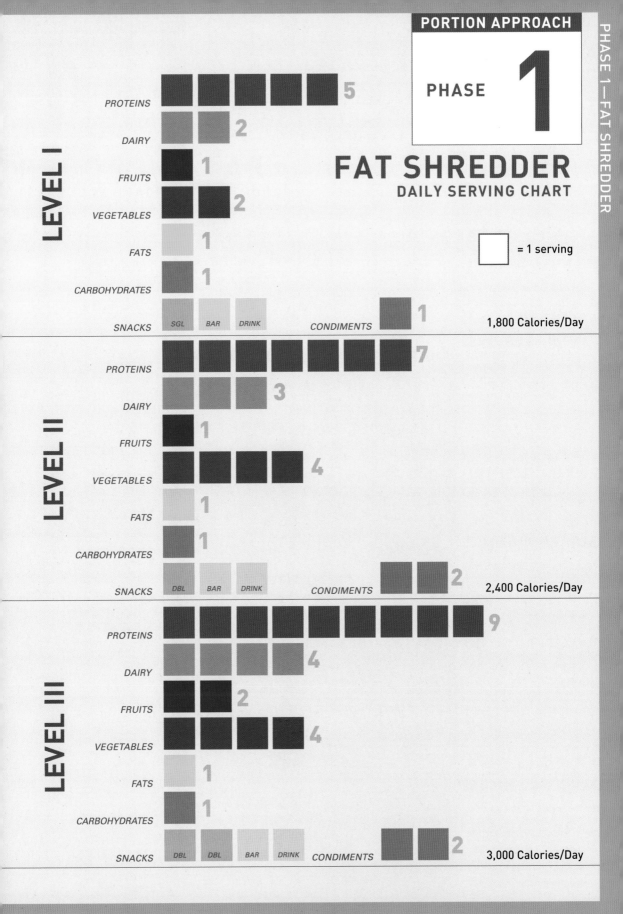

PORTION APPROACH

PHASE 1

FAT SHREDDER
DAILY SERVING CHART

= 1 serving

LEVEL I

PROTEINS 5
DAIRY 2
FRUITS 1
VEGETABLES 2
FATS 1
CARBOHYDRATES 1
SNACKS — SGL BAR DRINK — CONDIMENTS 1

1,800 Calories/Day

LEVEL II

PROTEINS 7
DAIRY 3
FRUITS 1
VEGETABLES 4
FATS 1
CARBOHYDRATES 1
SNACKS — DBL BAR DRINK — CONDIMENTS 2

2,400 Calories/Day

LEVEL III

PROTEINS 9
DAIRY 4
FRUITS 2
VEGETABLES 4
FATS 1
CARBOHYDRATES 1
SNACKS — DBL DBL BAR DRINK — CONDIMENTS 2

3,000 Calories/Day

During Phase 1, use the following list to determine which foods to purchase from the grocery store and what amount constitutes one serving. Remember, the foods you choose to incorporate in your diet are up to you—just make sure the portions fit within the parameters of your determined nutrition level.

FAT SHREDDER
PORTION APPROACH FOODS LIST

FATS

Each serving = 120 calories

3 oz._Avocado   Olive oil_1Tbsp.
1 Tbsp._Canola oil   Olives_4 oz.
1Tbsp._Flaxseed oil

PROTEINS

Each serving = 100 calories

3 oz._Boneless, skinless chicken or turkey breast	Soy burger_1
6_Egg whites	Soy cheese slices_5
3 oz._Fish and shellfish	Tofu_3 oz.
3 oz._Ham slices, fat-free	Tuna_3 oz.
3 oz._Pork tenderloin	Turkey bacon_2 slices
1/3 cup_Beachbody Whey Protein Powder	Veggie burger_1
3 oz._Red meat (top sirloin, flank steak)	Veggie dog_1
3 oz._Red meat, lean	

CARBOHYDRATES GRAINS LEGUMES POTATOES

Each serving = 200 calories

1 medium_Bagel, whole wheat	Pancakes (3.6 oz.)_3
1 cup_Baked beans	Pasta or noodles_1 cup
1 cup_Beans (kidney, black, etc.)	Pita, whole wheat_1 large
1_Bran muffin (2.5 oz)	Potato_1 medium
2 slices_Bread (whole wheat, rye, or pumpernickel)	Quinoa_1 cup
1 cup_Cereal, whole grain	Refried beans, low-fat_1 cup
1 cup_Couscous	Rice, brown or wild_1 cup
12_Crackers	Sweet potato_1 medium
2_ English muffin halves, whole wheat	Tortillas, corn_3
1 cup_Hummus	Tortilla, whole wheat_1 large
1 cup_Lentils	Waffles, whole wheat_2
1 cup_Oatmeal	Wheat berries_1 cup

DAIRY PRODUCTS

Each serving = 120 calories

Note: One portion of low-fat cheese or cottage cheese counts as either a snack or a dairy portion, not both.

1 oz._Cheese, low-fat	Parmesan cheese_1 oz.
1 cup_Cottage cheese, 1%	Skim milk_8 oz.
1 oz._Feta cheese	Soy cheese_1 oz.
1 oz._Goat cheese, semisoft	Soy milk_8 oz.
1-1/2 oz._Mozzarella, part-skim	Yogurt, plain nonfat_8 oz.

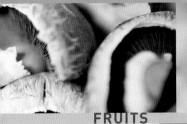

FRUITS

Each serving = 100 calories

1 medium_Apple	Nectarine_1 medium
1 cup_Apricots	Orange_1 large
1 medium_Banana	Papaya_1/2 medium
1/4 medium_Cantaloupe	Peach_1 medium
1 cup_Cherries	Pear_1 medium
1 oz._Dried fruit	Raspberries, blueberries, blackberries_1 cup
1 medium_Grapefruit	Strawberries, sliced_2 cups
1 cup_Grapes	Tangerine_1 medium
1 cup_Kiwi	Watermelon_1 cup
1/2 medium_Mango	

VEGETABLES

Each serving = 50 calories

1 serving = 1 cup cooked vegetables, vegetable juice, or vegetable soup

1 serving = 2 cups leafy greens

Asparagus	Kale
Beets	Lettuce
Bok choy	Marinara sauce
Broccoli	Mushrooms
Brussels sprouts	Peas
Cabbage	Peppers
Carrots	Spinach
Cauliflower	Sprouts
Celery	Squash (summer or winter)
Collard greens	String beans
Cucumber	Tomatoes
Eggplant	Vegetable soup

CONDIMENTS

Each serving = 50 calories (2 Tbsp.)

BBQ and other low-fat sauces and marinades, fat-free dressings, mustard, honey, pure fruit jams

SNACKS

Single serving = 100 calories

Double serving = 200 calories

Note: One portion of low-fat cheese or cottage cheese counts as either a snack or a dairy portion, not both.

Single	Double
1 oz._Cheese, low-fat	Cottage cheese, 1%_12 oz.
8 oz._Cottage cheese, 1%	Nuts_1 oz. (almonds, cashews, pecans, 30 pistachios)
1 oz._Dried fruit	
12_Mini rice cakes	P90X Peak Performance Protein Bar_1
1/2_P90X Peak Performance Protein Bar	P90X Results and Recovery Formula_12 to 16 oz.
1 Tbsp._Peanut butter with celery sticks	Soy nuts_4 oz.
2 oz._Soy nuts	String cheese_3 oz.
1-1/2 oz._String cheese	Turkey jerky_2 oz.
1 oz._Turkey jerky	
8 oz._Yogurt, plain nonfat	
2/3 scoop_Shakeology*	

*For more information on Shakeology, please refer to page 15.

SHAKEOLOGY

Single
2/3_serving for amount

PORTION APPROACH

PHASE 1

FAT SHREDDER

GENERAL GUIDELINES

Following the Meal Plan Approach will take the guesswork out of your daily food preparation. You'll enjoy a variety of delicious, healthy, low-fat recipes that'll provide you with the proper amount of nutrition and energy to get the most out of your P90X workout.

FAT SHREDDER

_Recipe included

	BREAKFAST	SNACK	LUNCH	SNACK	DINNER
DAY 1	1_Mushroom Omelet ▦ 1 cup_Fresh strawberries 8 oz._Cottage cheese, 1%	1_P90X Peak Performance Protein Bar 1_Results and Recovery Formula drink**	1_Chef Salad ▦	2 oz._Soy nuts	6 oz._Salmon 2 Tbsp._Lemon-Dill Sauce ▦ 1/2 cup_Asparagus 1 cup_Wild rice 1 cup_Red Pepper Soup ▦ 1 Tbsp._Beachbody Whey Protein Powder
DAY 2	1_Shakeology P90X-tra Shake* ▦ 1_Banana	1_P90X Peak Performance Protein Bar 1_Results and Recovery Formula drink**	1_Shrimp Stir-Fry ▦ 1 Tbsp._Sesame seeds 1 oz._Cashews	1-1/2 oz._String cheese	6 oz._Turkey 2 Tbsp._Gravy ▦ 1/2 cup_Green beans 1 cup_Butternut Squash Soup 1 Tbsp._Beachbody Whey Protein Powder
DAY 3	2 slices_Turkey bacon 1_Chicken Scramble ▦ 4 oz._Fresh-squeezed juice	1_P90X Peak Performance Protein Bar 1_Results and Recovery Formula drink**	1_Chicken Salad ▦ 2 cups_Salad greens 1 cup_Vegetable Soup ▦ 1 Tbsp._Beachbody Whey Protein Powder	2 oz._Soy nuts	6 oz._Halibut 2 Tbsp._Pesto Sauce ▦ 1 cup_Wild rice 1/2 cup_Zucchini
DAY 4	1_Soy Sausage Muffin ▦ 8 oz._Skim milk	1_P90X Peak Performance Protein Bar 1_Results and Recovery Formula drink**	1_Steak and Arugula Salad ▦ 2 Tbsp._Balsamic Vinaigrette ▦	1 oz._Turkey jerky	6 oz._Chicken breast 2 Tbsp._Honey-Chile Sauce ▦ 1 cup_Quinoa 1/2 cup_Snap peas
DAY 5	1_Spinach Scramble ▦ 8 oz._Skim milk 1/2_Grapefruit, medium	1_P90X Peak Performance Protein Bar 1_Results and Recovery Formula drink**	6 oz._Turkey Burger ▦ 1-1/2 oz._Low-fat Swiss cheese 1/2 cup_Coleslaw ▦ 1 cup_Gazpacho ▦ 1 Tbsp._Beachbody Whey Protein Powder	8 oz._Cottage cheese, 1%	6 oz._Swordfish 2 Tbsp._Mango-Ginger Sauce ▦ 1 cup_Wild rice 1_Artichoke, medium
DAY 6	1_Shakeology P90X-tra Shake* ▦ 1_Banana	1_P90X Peak Performance Protein Bar 1_Results and Recovery Formula drink**	1_Island Pork Tenderloin Salad ▦	1 oz._Turkey jerky	1_Beef and Broccoli Stir-Fry ▦ 1 cup_Miso Soup ▦ 1 Tbsp._Beachbody Whey Protein Powder
DAY 7	2 slices_Turkey bacon 1_Cheese Scramble ▦ 8 oz._Skim milk 1/4_Cantaloupe, medium	1_P90X Peak Performance Protein Bar 1_Results and Recovery Formula drink**	1_Tuna Salad ▦ 2 cups_Salad greens 1 cup_Chilled Cucumber Soup ▦	8 oz._Cottage cheese, 1%	6 oz_Lemon-Garlic Chicken ▦ 1 cup_Wild rice 1 cup_Asparagus Soup ▦ 1 Tbsp._Beachbody Whey Protein Powder

*For more information on Shakeology, please refer to page 15.

**Immediately after workout.

FAT SHREDDER

MEAL PLAN APPROACH

LEVEL II
PHASE 1

BREAKFAST	SNACK	LUNCH	SNACK	DINNER
1 1_Mushroom Omelet 1 cup_Fresh strawberries 12 oz._Cottage cheese, 1%	1_P90X Peak Performance Protein Bar 1_Results and Recovery Formula drink**	1_Chef Salad	30_Pistachio nuts	8 oz._Salmon 3 Tbsp._Lemon-Dill Sauce 1 cup_Asparagus 1 cup_Wild rice 2 cups_Red Pepper Soup 2 Tbsp._Beachbody Whey Protein Powder
2 1_Shakeology P90X-tra Shake* 1_Banana	1_P90X Peak Performance Protein Bar 1_Results and Recovery Formula drink**	1_Shrimp Stir-Fry 1 Tbsp._Sesame seeds 1 oz._Cashews	3 oz._String cheese	8 oz._Turkey 3 Tbsp._Gravy 1 cup_Green beans 2 cups_Butternut Squash Soup 2 Tbsp._Beachbody Whey Protein Powder
3 3 slices_Turkey bacon 1_Chicken Scramble 6 oz._Fresh-squeezed juice	1_P90X Peak Performance Protein Bar 1_Results and Recovery Formula drink**	1_Chicken Salad 3 cups_Salad greens 2 cups_Vegetable Soup 2 Tbsp._Beachbody Whey Protein Powder	4 oz._Soy nuts	8 oz._Halibut 3 Tbsp._Pesto Sauce 1 cup_Wild rice 1 cup_Zucchini
4 1_Soy Sausage Muffin 12 oz._Skim milk	1_P90X Peak Performance Protein Bar 1_Results and Recovery Formula drink**	1_Steak and Arugula Salad 3 Tbsp._Balsamic Vinaigrette	2 oz._Turkey jerky	8 oz._Chicken breast 3 Tbsp._Honey-Chile Sauce 1 cup_Quinoa 1 cup_Snap peas
5 1_Spinach Scramble 12 oz._Skim milk 1_Grapefruit, medium	1_P90X Peak Performance Protein Bar 1_Results and Recovery Formula drink**	8 oz._Turkey Burger 3 oz._Low-fat Swiss cheese 1/2 cup_Coleslaw 1 cup_Gazpacho 2 Tbsp._Beachbody Whey Protein Powder	12 oz._Cottage cheese, 1%	8 oz._Swordfish 3 Tbsp._Mango-Ginger Sauce 1 cup_Wild rice 1_Artichoke, medium
6 1_Shakeology P90X-tra Shake* 1_Banana	1_P90X Peak Performance Protein Bar 1_Results and Recovery Formula drink**	1_Island Pork Tenderloin Salad	2 oz._Turkey jerky	1_Beef and Broccoli Stir-Fry 2 cups_Miso Soup 2 Tbsp._Beachbody Whey Protein Powder
7 3 slices_Turkey bacon 1_Cheese Scramble 12 oz._Skim milk 1/4_Cantaloupe, medium	1_P90X Peak Performance Protein Bar 1_Results and Recovery Formula drink**	1_Tuna Salad 3 cups_Salad greens 2 cups_Chilled Cucumber Soup	12 oz._Cottage cheese, 1%	8 oz_Lemon-Garlic Chicken 1 cup_Wild rice 2 cups_Asparagus Soup 2 Tbsp._Beachbody Whey Protein Powder

*For more information on Shakeology, please refer to page 15.

**Immediately after workout.

FAT SHREDDER

_Recipe included

	BREAKFAST	SNACK	LUNCH	SNACK	DINNER
DAY 1	1_Mushroom Omelet 1 cup_Fresh strawberries 12 oz._Cottage cheese, 1%	1_P90X Peak Performance Protein Bar 1_Results and Recovery Formula drink**	1_Chef Salad	30_Pistachio nuts 2 oz._Turkey jerky	10 oz._Salmon 4 Tbsp._Lemon-Dill Sauce 1 cup_Asparagus 1 cup_Wild rice 2 cups_Red Pepper Soup 3 Tbsp._Beachbody Whey Protein Powder
DAY 2	1_Shakeology P90X-tra Shake*	1_P90X Peak Performance Protein Bar 1_Results and Recovery Formula drink**	1_Shrimp Stir-Fry 2 Tbsp._Sesame seeds 1 oz._Cashews	3 oz._String cheese 4 oz._Soy nuts	10 oz._Turkey 4 Tbsp._Gravy 1 cup_Green beans 2 cups_Butternut Squash Soup 3 Tbsp._Beachbody Whey Protein Powder
DAY 3	4 slices_Turkey bacon 1_Chicken Scramble 8 oz._Fresh-squeezed juice	1_P90X Peak Performance Protein Bar 1_Results and Recovery Formula drink**	1_Chicken Salad 4 cups_Salad greens 2 cups_Vegetable Soup 3 Tbsp._Beachbody Whey Protein Powder	4 oz._Soy nuts 12 oz._Cottage cheese, 1%	10 oz._Halibut 4 Tbsp._Pesto Sauce 1 cup_Wild rice 1 cup_Zucchini
DAY 4	1_Soy Sausage Muffin 12 oz._Skim milk	1_P90X Peak Performance Protein Bar 1_Results and Recovery Formula drink**	1_Steak and Arugula Salad 4 Tbsp._Balsamic Vinaigrette	3 oz._String Cheese 1 oz._Cashews	10 oz._Chicken breast 4 Tbsp._Honey-Chile Sauce 1 cup_Quinoa 1 cup_Snap peas
DAY 5	1_Spinach Scramble 12 oz._Skim milk 1_Grapefruit, medium	1_P90X Peak Performance Protein Bar 1_Results and Recovery Formula drink**	10 oz._Turkey Burger 3 oz._Low-fat Swiss cheese 2 cups_Coleslaw 2 cups_Gazpacho 3 Tbsp._Beachbody Whey Protein Powder	12 oz._Cottage cheese, 1% 2 oz._Turkey jerky	10 oz._Swordfish 4 Tbsp._Mango-Ginger Sauce 1 cup_Wild rice 1_Artichoke, medium
DAY 6	1_Shakeology P90X-tra Shake*	1_P90X Peak Performance Protein Bar 1_Results and Recovery Formula drink**	1_Island Pork Tenderloin Salad	2 oz._Turkey jerky 1 oz._Almonds	1_Beef and Broccoli Stir-Fry 2 cups_Miso Soup 3 Tbsp._Beachbody Whey Protein Powder
DAY 7	4 slices_Turkey bacon 1_Cheese Scramble 12 oz._Skim milk 1/2_Cantaloupe, medium	1_P90X Peak Performance Protein Bar 1_Results and Recovery Formula drink**	1_Tuna Salad 4 cups_Salad greens 2 cups_Chilled Cucumber Soup	12 oz._Cottage cheese, 1% 1 oz._Almonds	10 oz_Lemon-Garlic Chicken 1 cup_Wild rice 2 cups_Asparagus Soup 3 Tbsp._Beachbody Whey Protein Powder

*For more information on Shakeology, please refer to page 15.

**Immediately after workout

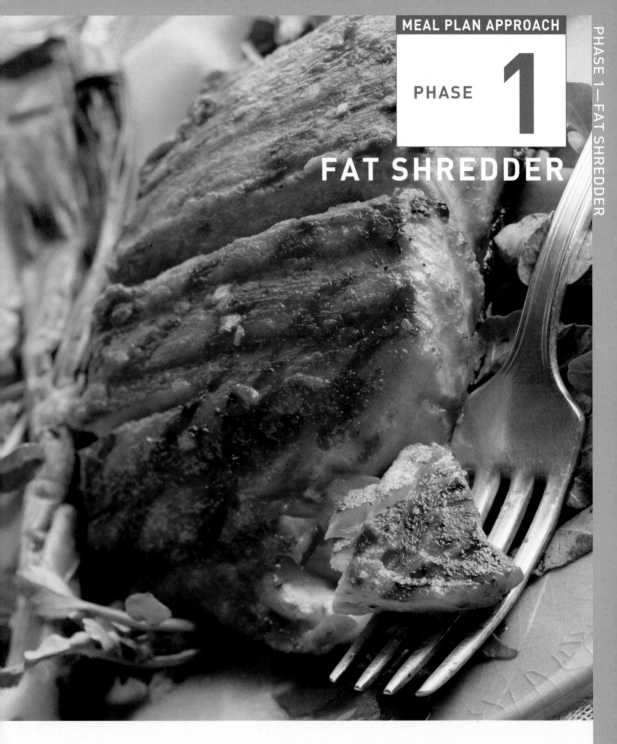

MEAL PLAN APPROACH

PHASE **1**

FAT SHREDDER

High in protein and fiber, these recipes will put you on the fast track toward building lean muscle mass while shedding excess body fat. From soup to stir-fry, there are plenty of delicious food options to help speed up your metabolism and give your body the fuel it needs for the new challenges that lie ahead.

GENERAL GUIDELINES

NOTE: All per-serving nutritional information is based on one LEVEL I serving. LEVEL II and LEVEL III will vary, depending on portion size.

BALSAMIC VINAIGRETTE

per serving:

3/4 cup balsamic vinegar
1 Tbsp. fresh lemon juice
3 Tbsp. Dijon mustard
2 tsp. chopped shallots
2 tsp. chopped fresh basil
1 tsp. olive oil
Black pepper to taste

Calories (kcal)..............**14**
Total Fat......................**1 g**
(42% calories from fat)
Protein ....**0 g**
Carbohydrate ....**2 g**
Cholesterol ....**0 mg**
Sodium...................**71 mg**

Serves 8

Whisk all ingredients together in a small bowl. Cover and store in refrigerator.

LEVEL I
2 Tbsp.=1 condiment

LEVEL II
3 Tbsp.=1-1/2 condiments

LEVEL III
4 Tbsp.=2 condiments

CUMIN VINAIGRETTE

per serving:

2 Tbsp. fresh lime juice
1/2 Tbsp. orange juice
1/2 Tbsp. Dijon mustard
1/2 tsp. ground cumin
1/4 tsp. salt
1/8 tsp. black pepper
1 Tbsp. olive oil

Calories (kcal)..............**69**
Total Fat......................**7 g**
(92% calories from fat)
Protein ....**0 g**
Carbohydrate ....**2 g**
Cholesterol ....**0 mg**
Sodium.................**329 mg**

Serves 2

Whisk together until well mixed.

LEVEL I
2 Tbsp.=1 condiment

LEVEL II
3 Tbsp.=1-1/2 condiments

LEVEL III
4 Tbsp.=2 condiments

PESTO SAUCE

per serving:

1/2 cup pine nuts
2 cups fresh basil, packed
1 Tbsp. chopped garlic
1/2 cup grated low-fat Parmesan cheese
3 Tbsp. white cooking wine
3 Tbsp. lemon juice
1/4 cup fat-free low-sodium chicken or vegetable broth
Salt (to taste)

Calories (kcal)............**67**	
Total Fat....................**6 g**	
(9% calories from fat)	
Protein ....**2 g**	
Carbohydrate ....**2 g**	
Cholesterol ....**4 mg**	
Sodium................ **137 mg**	

Serves 10

1. Heat skillet over medium-high heat and toast nuts, turning until golden brown.
2. In food processor, puree basil, toasted nuts, and garlic. Add Parmesan cheese, wine, lemon juice, and chicken broth and process until blended. Add salt to taste and blend. Serve on pasta, chicken, or seafood.

LEVEL I	LEVEL II	LEVEL III
2 Tbsp.=1 condiment	3 Tbsp.=1-1/2 condiments	4 Tbsp.=2 condiments

MANGO-GINGER SAUCE

per serving:

1/2 Tbsp. olive oil
1 cup finely chopped red onion
1 cup peeled, cubed mango
1/2 cup chopped tomato
1-1/2 Tbsp. minced fresh ginger
1/4 cup fresh lime juice
2 Tbsp. orange juice
2 Tbsp. dry sherry
1-1/2 Tbsp. brown sugar
1-1/2 Tbsp. white vinegar

Calories (kcal)..............**46**	
Total Fat.....................**1 g**	
(19% calories from fat)	
Protein ....**1 g**	
Carbohydrate ....**9 g**	
Cholesterol ....**0 mg**	
Sodium....................**3 mg**	

Serves 8

Stir together all ingredients in a nonreactive bowl. Store covered in refrigerator until ready to serve.

LEVEL I	LEVEL II	LEVEL III
2 Tbsp.=1 condiment	3 Tbsp.=1-1/2 condiments	4 Tbsp.=2 condiments

GRAVY

1/3 cup chopped shallots
  1/3 cup all-purpose flour
    3 cups fat-free low-sodium chicken broth
      1/4 tsp. salt
        1 tsp. poultry seasoning

Calories (kcal)	**34**
Total Fat	**‹1 g**
(1% calories from fat)	
Protein	**4 g**
Carbohydrate	**4 g**
Cholesterol	**0 mg**
Sodium	**229 mg**

Serves 10

1. Sauté shallots in some of the broth until soft (see Low-Fat Cooking Techniques). Gradually whisk in the flour, adding broth as needed to form a thick paste.
2. Gradually add remaining broth, stirring and cooking until thickened. Add salt and poultry seasoning.

LEVEL I	**LEVEL II**	**LEVEL III**
2 Tbsp.=1 condiment	3 Tbsp.=1-1/2 condiments	4 Tbsp.=2 condiments

HONEY-CHILE SAUCE

1/4 cup finely chopped shallots
  2/3 cup honey, slightly warmed
    1/4 cup sherry vinegar
      1 tsp. pasilla chile powder
        1/4 tsp. ground cumin
          1-1/2 cups fat-free low-sodium chicken or vegetable broth
            Salt and pepper (to taste)
              1 tsp. chopped cilantro
                3 Tbsp. chopped pecans, toasted

Calories (kcal)	**56**
Total Fat	**1 g**
(13% calories from fat)	
Protein	**1 g**
Carbohydrate	**13 g**
Cholesterol	**0 mg**
Sodium	**48 mg**

Serves 16

1. Lightly coat a sauté pan with cooking spray and place over medium-high heat. Add shallots and sauté until tender.
2. Add honey and vinegar to pan. Quickly stir in chile powder, cumin, and broth. Bring to a boil and boil until reduced by half.
3. Transfer sauce to a blender or food processor and blend at high speed until smooth. Season to taste with salt and pepper. Stir in cilantro. Garnish dish with toasted pecans.

LEVEL I	**LEVEL II**	**LEVEL III**
2 Tbsp.=1 condiment	3 Tbsp.=1-1/2 condiments	4 Tbsp.=2 condiments

LEMON-DILL SAUCE

per serving:

1/2 cup chopped shallots

2 cups white wine

2 Tbsp. arrowroot powder

2 cups fat-free low-sodium chicken broth

6 Tbsp. lemon juice

1 tsp. minced lemongrass

1 Tbsp. chopped fresh dill

Calories (kcal)..............**58**

Total Fat....................**‹1 g**

(0% calories from fat)

Protein ....**3 g**

Carbohydrate ....**5 g**

Cholesterol ....**0 mg**

Sodium ....**107 mg**

Serves 10

1. Coat a large sauté pan with cooking spray; sauté shallots until soft (not brown), moistening with wine if necessary.
2. In a medium bowl, dissolve arrowroot in 1/2 cup of chicken broth and set aside.
3. Add remaining wine to shallots, bring to boil, and boil until reduced by half. Add remaining chicken broth, return to boil, and reduce by half again.
4. Add arrowroot mixture to pan and stir to blend. Transfer contents to a food processor or blender and puree until smooth.
5. Return sauce to pan. Add lemon juice and lemongrass and simmer over low heat for about 30 minutes, until thick. Strain out lemongrass and stir in dill.

LEVEL I	LEVEL II	LEVEL III
2 Tbsp.=1 condiment	3 Tbsp.=1-1/2 condiments	4 Tbsp.=2 condiments

CHILLED CUCUMBER SOUP

per serving:

1 whole cucumber

1/2 cup chopped red onion

3 Tbsp. chopped fresh dill

1 Tbsp. chopped fresh mint

1-1/4 cups nonfat plain yogurt

1/4 tsp. salt

1/8 tsp. black pepper

1/16 tsp. cayenne pepper

1/4 Tbsp. celery seed

Calories (kcal)..............**60**

Total Fat....................**‹1 g**

(5% calories from fat)

Protein ....**5 g**

Carbohydrate ....**10 g**

Cholesterol ....**1 mg**

Sodium ....**191 mg**

Serves 4

Combine all ingredients in blender and puree. Chill. Garnish with chopped dill or parsley.

LEVEL I	LEVEL II	LEVEL III
1 cup soup =1/2 vegetable	2 cups soup =1 vegetable	3 cups soup =1-1/2 vegetables

ASPARAGUS SOUP

per serving:

1-1/4 cups diced onions

1/2 tsp. chopped garlic

1-1/2 quarts fat-free low-sodium chicken or vegetable broth

1-1/2 pounds asparagus, diced

1/2 potato, diced

1 dash salt

1/2 tsp. yellow mustard seed

1 dash 17-spice mix

1/2 tsp. dry mustard

Calories (kcal).............**38**	
Total Fat....................**<1 g**	
(0% calories from fat)	
Protein ....**2 g**	
Carbohydrate ....**5 g**	
Cholesterol ....**0 mg**	
Sodium............. **1,780 mg**	

Serves 8

1. Sauté onions and garlic in 1/4 cup of chicken broth.

2. Add asparagus, potato, and remaining broth. Bring to a boil. Reduce heat and simmer 15 to 20 minutes.

3. Remove soup from heat and puree with a food processor or immersion blender. Return to pan and season with spices.

4. Serve.

LEVEL I	LEVEL II	LEVEL III
1 cup soup = 1 vegetable	2 cups soup = 2 vegetables	3 cups soup = 3 vegetables

BUTTERNUT SQUASH SOUP

per serving:

1 Tbsp. minced shallot

1 clove garlic, pressed or minced

3 cups cubed butternut squash

1/2 cup fat-free low-sodium chicken or vegetable broth

Calories (kcal).............**70**	
Total Fat....................**<1 g**	
(1% calories from fat)	
Protein ....**3 g**	
Carbohydrate ....**18 g**	
Cholesterol ....**0 mg**	
Sodium..................**89 mg**	

Serves 3

1. Place shallot and garlic in a nonstick saucepan and cook over low heat until translucent, adding a little water if necessary to prevent scorching.

2. Add chicken broth and bring to a simmer. Add squash and simmer until squash is soft, about 20 minutes. Transfer to a blender or food processor and puree.

3. Return soup to pan and place over medium heat until heated through.

4. Serve.

LEVEL I	LEVEL II	LEVEL III
1 cup soup = 1 vegetable	2 cups soup = 3 vegetables	2 cups soup = 3 vegetables

GAZPACHO

per serving:

14 oz. canned low-sodium tomatoes
1-1/2 cups low-sodium tomato juice
1-1/4 cups peeled, diced cucumbers
1/4 cup peeled, diced carrots
1/2 cup each diced green and red bell pepper
1/2 red onion, diced
1 shallot, peeled
1 garlic clove, peeled
3 Tbsp. red wine vinegar
3 Tbsp. fresh lemon juice
1/2 tsp. paprika
2 Tbsp. each chopped fresh oregano, basil, and Italian parsley
1/8 tsp. white pepper
Tabasco® sauce (to taste)

Calories (kcal)	20
Total Fat	‹1 g
(4% calories from fat)	
Protein	1 g
Carbohydrate	5 g
Cholesterol	0 mg
Sodium	5 mg

Serves 5

1. Place tomatoes, tomato juice, cucumbers, carrots, peppers, onion, shallots, and garlic in
   a food processor or blender and process until smooth.

2. Add vinegar, lemon juice, paprika, oregano, basil, parsley, and white pepper and process to combine.
   Add Tabasco sauce to taste and blend. Chill for several hours before serving.

LEVEL I
1 cup soup = 1/2 vegetable

LEVEL II
2 cups soup = 1 vegetable

LEVEL III
3 cups soup = 1-1/2 vegetables

MISO SOUP

per serving:

1/2 teaspoon dark sesame oil
1/3 cup finely chopped shallots
3 Tbsp. miso
1 quart vegetable stock
1/4 cup diced firm silken tofu
3 Tbsp. sliced scallions (for garnish)

Calories (kcal)	107
Total Fat	3 g
(23% calories from fat)	
Protein	4 g
Carbohydrate	16 g
Cholesterol	1 mg
Sodium	1,052 mg

Serves 8

1. Heat sesame oil in a saucepan over medium heat. Add shallots and cook until translucent.

2. Add miso and mix well. Add stock and bring to a simmer. Reduce heat to low and simmer for 15 minutes.

3. To serve, ladle into bowls and garnish each serving with tofu and scallions.

4. Serve.

LEVEL I
1 cup soup = 1 vegetable, 1/2 protein

LEVEL II
2 cups soup = 2 vegetables, 1 protein

LEVEL III
3 cups soup = 3 vegetables,
1-1/2 protein

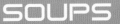

SOUPS

33

VEGETABLE SOUP

10 cups fat-free low-sodium chicken or vegetable broth

4 medium red potatoes, cut into 1-inch cubes

4 cups quartered onions

1 cup sliced carrots (1 inch thick)

3 cups sliced celery (1 inch thick)

2 cups sliced zucchini (1 inch thick)

8 ounces canned tomato sauce

2 cloves garlic, minced

1/4 bunch fresh parsley, chopped

1/4 bunch cilantro, chopped

Serves 18

1 dash black pepper

Calories (kcal)..............**49**	
Total Fat.....................**‹1 g**	
(2% calories from fat)	
Protein ....**7 g**	
Carbohydrate ....**10 g**	
Cholesterol ....**0 mg**	
Sodium.................**377 mg**	

1. In a large stockpot, combine chicken broth, potatoes, onions, carrots, and celery. Bring to a boil, then reduce heat to medium-high and simmer until potatoes are tender, about 30 minutes.

2. Add zucchini, tomato sauce, garlic, parsley, and cilantro. Reduce heat to medium-low and cook for 10 to 15 minutes more, or until zucchini is just tender. Season to taste with black pepper and serve.

LEVEL I	LEVEL II	LEVEL III
1 cup soup = 1 vegetable	2 cups soup = 2 vegetables	3 cups soup = 3 vegetables

RED PEPPER SOUP

2 cups white wine (more if needed)

1 onion, finely chopped

5 roasted red peppers, cored, seeded, and chopped

2 cups chopped celery

1 Tbsp. minced garlic

2 plum tomatoes, chopped

1/4 cup tomato paste

2 cups fat-free low-sodium chicken or vegetable broth

2 Tbsp. dried thyme

1/4 tsp. each ground white pepper and ground cumin

Serves 12

1 dash salt

Calories (kcal)..............**57**	
Total Fat.....................**‹1 g**	
(5% calories from fat)	
Protein ....**3 g**	
Carbohydrate ....**6 g**	
Cholesterol ....**0 mg**	
Sodium.................**145 mg**	

1. Heat wine in a large, heavy soup pot over medium heat. Add onion, red peppers, and celery. Cook and stir for 3 minutes. Stir in garlic. Cook for 2 more minutes, adding more wine if necessary.

2. Add tomatoes, tomato paste, and broth; cover and bring to a boil. Reduce heat and simmer for 25 minutes.

3. Puree soup in a food processor or blender. Return to the pan, add seasonings, and heat through.

4. Serve.

LEVEL I	LEVEL II	LEVEL III
1 cup soup = 1 vegetable	2 cups soup = 2 vegetables	3 cups soup = 3 vegetables

SHAKEOLOGY P90X-TRA—LEVEL I

per serving:

3/4 cup nonfat milk
1/2 cup water
1 scoop Chocolate Shakeology
1/2 cup berries
1/2 small banana
1/2 cup ice

Calories (kcal)	**289**
Total Fat	**2 g**
(6% calories from fat)	
Protein	**25 g**
Carbohydrate	**45 g**
Cholesterol	**19 mg**
Sodium	**178 mg**

1. Add milk, water, Shakeology, berries, banana, and ice to blender. Blend until smooth.
2. Serve immediately.

LEVEL I	LEVEL II	LEVEL III
1 protein, 1 dairy, 1 fruit	See below	See next page

SHAKEOLOGY P90X-TRA—LEVEL II

per serving:

1 cup nonfat milk
1-1/2 scoops Chocolate Shakeology
1/2 cup berries
1/2 small banana
1/2 cup ice

Calories (kcal)	**385**
Total Fat	**2 g**
(6% calories from fat)	
Protein	**37 g**
Carbohydrate	**57 g**
Cholesterol	**27 mg**
Sodium	**254 mg**

1. Add milk, Shakeology, berries, banana, and ice to blender. Blend until smooth.
2. Serve immediately.

*For more information on Shakeology, please refer to page 15.

LEVEL I	LEVEL II	LEVEL III
See above	1-1/2 protein, 1 dairy, 1 fruit	See next page

SHAKEOLOGY P90X-TRA—LEVEL III

per serving:

1 cup nonfat milk

2 scoops Chocolate Shakeology

1 cup berries

1/2 small banana

1 cup ice

Calories (kcal)............**492**

Total Fat.....................**3 g**

(6% calories from fat)

Protein ....**46 g**

Carbohydrate ....**72 g**

Cholesterol ....**35 mg**

Sodium.................**305 mg**

1. Add milk, Shakeology, berries, banana, and ice to blender. Blend until smooth.
2. Serve immediately.

*For more information on Shakeology, please refer to page 15.

LEVEL I	LEVEL II	LEVEL III
See previous page	See previous page	2 protein, 1 dairy, 1-1/2 fruit

SOY SAUSAGE MUFFIN

per serving:

2 to 4 soy sausage patties (approximately 80 calories each)

1 to 2 whole wheat English muffins

1-1/2 to 4 oz. fat-free mozzarella cheese

Calories (kcal)..............**57**

Total Fat.....................**‹1 g**

(5% calories from fat)

Protein ....**3 g**

Carbohydrate ....**6 g**

Cholesterol ....**0 mg**

Sodium.................**145 mg**

1. Cook soy sausage according to package instructions.
2. Toast English muffin(s), then top with cheese and melt in toaster oven or under broiler for 2 to 3 minutes.
3. Place sausage on one muffin half and top with other half.

LEVEL I	LEVEL II	LEVEL III
2 soy patties, 1 English muffin, 1-1/2 oz. cheese = 1 protein, 1 carbohydrate, 1 dairy	3 soy patties, 1 English muffin, 3 oz. cheese = 2 protein, 1 carbohydrate, 2 dairy	4 soy patties, 2 English muffins, 4 oz. cheese = 3 protein, 2 carbohydrate, 2 dairy

CHICKEN SCRAMBLE—LEVEL I

per serving:

6 egg whites
   3 oz. chicken breast, cooked and diced
     1 oz. feta cheese, crumbled
       1-1/2 Tbsp. chopped fresh basil
         Salt and pepper (to taste)

Calories (kcal)	**308**
Total Fat	**9 g**
(14% calories from fat)	
Protein	**52 g**
Carbohydrate	**3 g**
Cholesterol	**96 mg**
Sodium	**703 mg**

1. Lightly coat a nonstick skillet with cooking spray and place over medium heat.
2. Lightly beat egg whites with a fork and pour into pan. Cook, stirring, until halfway set. Add chicken and finish cooking until eggs are cooked through.
3. Place on plate. Salt and pepper to taste. Sprinkle with feta and garnish with basil.

LEVEL I
2 protein, 1 dairy

LEVEL II
See below

LEVEL III
See next page

CHICKEN SCRAMBLE—LEVEL II

per serving:

8 egg whites
   4 oz. chicken breast, cooked and diced
     1-1/2 oz. feta cheese, crumbled
       2 Tbsp. chopped fresh basil
         Salt and pepper (to taste)

Calories (kcal)	**424**
Total Fat	**13 g**
(21% calories from fat)	
Protein	**70 g**
Carbohydrate	**4 g**
Cholesterol	**133 mg**
Sodium	**990 mg**

1. Lightly coat a nonstick skillet with cooking spray and place over medium heat.
2. Lightly beat egg whites with a fork and pour into pan. Cook, stirring, until halfway set. Add chicken and finish cooking until eggs are cooked through.
3. Place on plate. Salt and pepper to taste. Sprinkle with feta and garnish with basil.

LEVEL I
See above

LEVEL II
2-1/2 protein, 1-1/2 dairy

LEVEL III
See next page

CHICKEN SCRAMBLE—LEVEL III

per serving:

10 egg whites
     5 oz. chicken breast, cooked and diced
       2 oz. feta cheese, crumbled
         3 Tbsp. chopped fresh basil
           Salt and pepper (to taste)

Calories (kcal)	**539**
Total Fat	**18 g**
(27% calories from fat)	
Protein	**88 g**
Carbohydrate	**5 g**
Cholesterol	**169 mg**
Sodium	**1,277 mg**

1. Lightly coat a nonstick skillet with cooking spray and place over medium heat.
2. Lightly beat egg whites with a fork and pour into pan. Cook, stirring, until halfway set. Add chicken and finish cooking until eggs are cooked through.
3. Place on plate. Salt and pepper to taste. Sprinkle with feta and garnish with basil.

LEVEL I	LEVEL II	LEVEL III
See previous page	See previous page	3 protein, 2 dairy

CHEESE SCRAMBLE—LEVEL I

per serving:

6 egg whites
     2 Tbsp. skim milk
       1-1/2 oz. part-skim mozzarella cheese, grated
         Salt and pepper (to taste)

Calories (kcal)	**230**
Total Fat	**4 g**
(29% calories from fat)	
Protein	**34 g**
Carbohydrate	**5 g**
Cholesterol	**24 mg**
Sodium	**450 mg**

1. Lightly coat a medium nonstick skillet with cooking spray and place over medium heat.
2. In a bowl, lightly beat egg whites with skim milk.
3. Pour egg mixture into pan and cook slightly, then add cheese and cook to desired firmness.

LEVEL I	LEVEL II	LEVEL III
1-1/2 protein, 1/2 dairy	See next page	See next page

CHEESE SCRAMBLE—LEVEL II

per serving:

8 egg whites
   3 Tbsp. skim milk
      3 oz. part-skim mozzarella cheese, grated
         Salt and pepper (to taste)

Calories (kcal)...........**388**
Total Fat....................**7 g**
(35% calories from fat)
Protein ....**53 g**
Carbohydrate ....**8 g**
Cholesterol ....**47 mg**
Sodium.................**653 mg**

1. Lightly coat a medium nonstick skillet with cooking spray and place over medium heat.
2. In a bowl, lightly beat egg whites with skim milk.
3. Pour egg mixture into pan and cook slightly, then add cheese and cook to desired firmness.

LEVEL I
See previous page

LEVEL II
2-1/2 protein, 1 dairy

LEVEL III
See below

CHEESE SCRAMBLE—LEVEL III

per serving:

10 egg whites
   4 Tbsp. skim milk
      4 oz. part-skim mozzarella cheese, grated
         Salt and pepper (to taste)

Calories (kcal)...........**506**
Total Fat....................**9 g**
(35% calories from fat)
Protein ....**68 g**
Carbohydrate ....**10 g**
Cholesterol ....**62 mg**
Sodium.................**845 mg**

1. Lightly coat a medium nonstick skillet with cooking spray and place over medium heat.
2. In a bowl, lightly beat egg whites with skim milk.
3. Pour egg mixture into pan and cook slightly, then add cheese and cook to desired firmness.

LEVEL I
See previous page

LEVEL II
See above

LEVEL III
3-1/2 protein, 1 dairy

SPINACH SCRAMBLE—LEVEL I

1/2 cup diced Roma tomatoes

    1 cup spinach leaves, cleaned and dried

        6 egg whites

            1-1/2 oz. feta cheese, crumbled

                1 Tbsp. chopped fresh basil

Calories (kcal)	**239**
Total Fat	**9 g**
(35% calories from fat)	
Protein	**29 g**
Carbohydrate	**9 g**
Cholesterol	**38 mg**
Sodium	**835 mg**

1. Place a small nonstick pan lightly coated with vegetable spray over medium heat. Sauté tomatoes and spinach until slightly tender. Place in separate dish and set aside.
2. Whisk egg whites together in a bowl and pour into pan. Cook, stirring, over low heat until almost set. Add vegetable mixture, cheese, and basil. Cook to desired firmness.

LEVEL I	LEVEL II	LEVEL III
1 protein, 1 dairy, 1 vegetable	See below	See next page

SPINACH SCRAMBLE—LEVEL II

1/2 cup diced Roma tomatoes

    1 cup spinach leaves, cleaned and dried

        8 egg whites

            3 oz. feta cheese, crumbled

                1 Tbsp. chopped fresh basil

Calories (kcal)	**384**
Total Fat	**18 g**
(43% calories from fat)	
Protein	**42 g**
Carbohydrate	**12 g**
Cholesterol	**76 mg**
Sodium	**1,419 mg**

1. Place a small nonstick pan lightly coated with vegetable spray over medium heat. Sauté tomatoes and spinach until slightly tender. Place in separate dish and set aside.
2. Whisk egg whites together in a bowl and pour into pan. Cook, stirring, over low heat until almost set. Add vegetable mixture, cheese, and basil. Cook to desired firmness.

LEVEL I	LEVEL II	LEVEL III
See above	1-1/2 protein, 1-1/2 dairy, 1 vegetable	See next page

BREAKFAST

SPINACH SCRAMBLE—LEVEL III

per serving:

1 cup diced Roma tomatoes

2 cups spinach leaves, cleaned and dried

10 egg whites

4 oz. feta cheese, crumbled

2 Tbsp. chopped fresh basil

Calories (kcal)............**518**

Total Fat....................**25 g**

(43% calories from fat)

Protein ....**55 g**

Carbohydrate ....**19 g**

Cholesterol ....**101 mg**

Sodium ....**1,877 mg**

1. Place a small nonstick pan lightly coated with vegetable spray over medium heat. Sauté tomatoes and spinach until slightly tender. Place in separate dish and set aside.
2. Whisk egg whites together in a bowl and pour into pan. Cook, stirring, over low heat until almost set. Add vegetable mixture, cheese, and basil. Cook to desired firmness.

LEVEL I

See previous page

LEVEL II

See previous page

LEVEL III

2 protein, 2 dairy, 2 vegetables

MUSHROOM OMELET—LEVEL I

per serving:

6 egg whites

Salt and pepper (to taste)

3/4 cup sliced mushrooms

2 Tbsp. chopped green onion

1/2 Roma tomato, chopped

1-1/2 oz. low-fat cheddar cheese, shredded

Calories (kcal)............**506**

Total Fat.....................**9 g**

(35% calories from fat)

Protein ....**68 g**

Carbohydrate ....**10 g**

Cholesterol ....**62 mg**

Sodium ....**845 mg**

1. In a small bowl, lightly beat egg whites with a fork and season to taste with salt and pepper.
2. Lightly coat a small nonstick sauté pan with cooking spray and place over medium heat. Add mushrooms, tomatoes, and green onion and cook until tender.
3. Add egg mixture and cook until set on the bottom. Sprinkle cheese over top, fold omelet in half, and cook a bit longer until cheese is melted and eggs are set. Serve.

LEVEL I

1 protein, 1/2 dairy, 1 vegetable

LEVEL II

See next page

LEVEL III

See next page

MUSHROOM OMELET—LEVEL II

8 egg whites

    Salt and pepper (to taste)

       3/4 cup sliced mushrooms

          2 Tbsp. chopped green onion

            1/2 Roma tomato, chopped

              3 oz. low-fat cheddar cheese, shredded

Calories (kcal)	**298**
Total Fat	**6 g**
(19% calories from fat)	
Protein	**50 g**
Carbohydrate	**8 g**
Cholesterol	**18 mg**
Sodium	**966 mg**

1. In a small bowl, lightly beat egg whites with a fork and season to taste with salt and pepper.
2. Lightly coat a small nonstick sauté pan with cooking spray and place over medium heat. Add mushrooms, tomatoes, and green onion and cook until tender.
3. Add egg mixture and cook until set on the bottom. Sprinkle cheese over top, fold omelet in half, and cook a bit longer until cheese is melted and eggs are set. Serve.

LEVEL I
See previous page

LEVEL II
1-1/2 protein, 1 dairy, 1 vegetable

LEVEL III
See below

MUSHROOM OMELET—LEVEL III

10 egg whites

    Salt and pepper (to taste)

       1 cup sliced mushrooms

          2 Tbsp. chopped green onion

            1/2 Roma tomato, chopped

              4 oz. low-fat cheddar cheese, shredded

Calories (kcal)	**395**
Total Fat	**8 g**
(19% calories from fat)	
Protein	**64 g**
Carbohydrate	**13 g**
Cholesterol	**24 mg**
Sodium	**1,256 mg**

1. In a small bowl, lightly beat egg whites with a fork and season to taste with salt and pepper.
2. Lightly coat a small nonstick sauté pan with cooking spray and place over medium heat. Add mushrooms, tomatoes, and green onion and cook until tender.
3. Add egg mixture and cook until set on the bottom. Sprinkle cheese over top, fold omelet in half, and cook a bit longer until cheese is melted and eggs are set. Serve.

LEVEL I
See previous page

LEVEL II
See above

LEVEL III
1-1/2 protein, 1-1/2 dairy, 1 vegetable

CHEF SALAD—LEVEL I

per serving:

3 oz. fat-free turkey breast, chopped

3 oz. extra-lean low-sodium ham, chopped

1-1/2 oz. fat-free mozzarella cheese, chopped

1/2 Roma tomato, chopped

2 cups chopped romaine lettuce

1/4 cup chopped hearts of palm

1 oz. avocado, diced

2 Tbsp. low-fat ranch dressing

Calories (kcal)............**323**
Total Fat.....................**8 g**
(21% calories from fat)
Protein ....**50 g**
Carbohydrate ....**14 g**
Cholesterol ....**86 mg**
Sodium.................**515 mg**

Toss all ingredients except dressing together in a bowl; drizzle with dressing.

LEVEL I
2 protein, 1/2 dairy, 2 vegetables,
1 condiment

LEVEL II
See below

LEVEL III
See next page

CHEF SALAD—LEVEL II

per serving:

4 oz. fat-free turkey breast, chopped

4 oz. extra-lean low-sodium ham, chopped

3 oz. fat-free mozzarella cheese, chopped

1/2 Roma tomato, chopped

2 cups chopped romaine lettuce

1/4 cup chopped hearts of palm

1 oz. avocado, diced

3 Tbsp. low-fat ranch dressing

Calories (kcal)............**452**
Total Fat.....................**9 g**
(18% calories from fat)
Protein ....**74 g**
Carbohydrate ....**18 g**
Cholesterol ....**119 mg**
Sodium.................**720 mg**

Toss all ingredients except dressing together in a bowl; drizzle with dressing.

LEVEL I
See above

LEVEL II
2-1/2 protein, 1 dairy, 2 vegetables,
1 condiment

LEVEL III
See next page

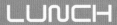

CHEF SALAD—LEVEL III

per serving:

5 oz. fat-free turkey breast, chopped

5 oz. extra-lean low-sodium ham, chopped

4 oz. fat-free mozzarella cheese, chopped

1 Roma tomato, chopped

2-1/2 cups chopped romaine lettuce

1/4 cup chopped hearts of palm

2 oz. avocado, diced

4 Tbsp. low-fat ranch dressing

Calories (kcal)	**611**
Total Fat	**14 g**
(20% calories from fat)	
Protein	**96 g**
Carbohydrate	**26 g**
Cholesterol	**150 mg**
Sodium	**913 mg**

Toss all ingredients except dressing together in a bowl; drizzle with dressing.

LEVEL I
See previous page

LEVEL II
See previous page

LEVEL III
3 protein, 2 dairy, 1 vegetable, 1 condiment

STEAK AND ARUGULA SALAD—LEVEL I

per serving:

6 oz. top sirloin

2 cups arugula

1/2 pint cherry tomatoes, halved

1/2 cup canned artichoke hearts, drained

2 Tbsp. Balsamic Vinaigrette (see recipe in Dressings)

Calories (kcal)	**398**
Total Fat	**11 g**
(42% calories from fat)	
Protein	**38 g**
Carbohydrate	**20 g**
Cholesterol	**87 mg**
Sodium	**293 mg**

1. Grill or broil steak until done, approximately 7 to 10 minutes on each side. Cool and cut into 1-inch slices.

2. Toss together arugula, tomatoes, and artichoke hearts and arrange on plates. Top with steak and drizzle with balsamic vinaigrette.

LEVEL I
2 protein, 3 vegetables, 1 condiment

LEVEL II
See next page

LEVEL III
See next page

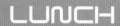

STEAK AND ARUGULA SALAD—LEVEL II

per serving:

8 oz. top sirloin

    3 cups arugula

        1/2 pint cherry tomatoes, halved

            3/4 cup canned artichoke hearts, drained

                3 Tbsp. Balsamic Vinaigrette (see recipe in Dressings)

Calories (kcal)	**531**
Total Fat	**14 g**
(42% calories from fat)	
Protein	**51 g**
Carbohydrate	**26 g**
Cholesterol	**116 mg**
Sodium	**414 mg**

1. Grill or broil steak until done, approximately 7 to 10 minutes on each side. Cool and cut into 1-inch slices.
2. Toss together arugula, tomatoes, and artichoke hearts and arrange on plates. Top with steak and drizzle with balsamic vinaigrette.

LEVEL I	LEVEL II	LEVEL III
See previous page	3 protein, 4 vegetables, 1 condiment	See below

STEAK AND ARUGULA SALAD—LEVEL III

per serving:

10 oz. top sirloin

    4 cups arugula

        1 pint cherry tomatoes, halved

            1 cup canned artichoke hearts, drained

                4 Tbsp. Balsamic Vinaigrette (see recipe in Dressings)

Calories (kcal)	**695**
Total Fat	**17 g**
(41% calories from fat)	
Protein	**66 g**
Carbohydrate	**40 g**
Cholesterol	**144 mg**
Sodium	**547 mg**

1. Grill or broil steak until done, approximately 7 to 10 minutes on each side. Cool and cut into 1-inch slices.
2. Toss together arugula, tomatoes, and artichoke hearts and arrange on plates. Top with steak and drizzle with balsamic vinaigrette.

LEVEL I	LEVEL II	LEVEL III
See previous page	See above	3-1/2 protein, 5 vegetables, 2 condiments

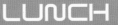

TUNA SALAD—LEVEL I

per serving:

6 oz. tuna canned in water, drained
1-1/2 Tbsp. low-fat mayonnaise
1/2 tsp. lemon zest
1 squeeze of fresh lemon juice
1 Tbsp. shredded carrots
1 Tbsp. chopped celery
1 Tbsp. chopped green onion
1 tsp. celery seeds

Calories (kcal)............**248**	
Total Fat....................**5 g**	
(17% calories from fat)	
Protein ....**44 g**	
Carbohydrate ....**5 g**	
Cholesterol ....**51 mg**	
Sodium.................**348 mg**	

Place tuna in a small bowl. Add mayonnaise and mix thoroughly. Then add lemon zest, lemon juice, carrots, celery, green onions, and celery seeds. Blend together. Serve.

LEVEL I	LEVEL II	LEVEL III
2 protein, 1 condiment	See below	See next page

TUNA SALAD—LEVEL II

per serving:

8 oz. tuna canned in water, drained
2 Tbsp. low-fat mayonnaise
1/2 tsp. lemon zest
1 squeeze of fresh lemon juice
2 Tbsp. shredded carrots
2 Tbsp. chopped celery
2 Tbsp. chopped green onion
1-1/2 tsp. celery seeds

Calories (kcal)............**337**	
Total Fat....................**7 g**	
(17% calories from fat)	
Protein ....**59 g**	
Carbohydrate ....**8 g**	
Cholesterol ....**68 mg**	
Sodium.................**447 mg**	

Place tuna in a small bowl. Add mayonnaise and mix thoroughly. Then add lemon zest, lemon juice, carrots, celery, green onions, and celery seeds. Blend together. Serve.

LEVEL I	LEVEL II	LEVEL III
See above	2-1/2 protein, 1 vegetable, 1 condiment	See next page

TUNA SALAD—LEVEL III

per serving:

10 oz. tuna canned in water, drained
2-1/2 Tbsp. low-fat mayonnaise
1 tsp. lemon zest
1 squeeze of fresh lemon juice
3 Tbsp. shredded carrots
3 Tbsp. chopped celery
3 Tbsp. chopped green onion
2 tsp. celery seeds

Calories (kcal)...........**459**
Total Fat..................**10 g**
(20% calories from fat)
Protein ....**75 g**
Carbohydrate ....**15 g**
Cholesterol ....**85 mg**
Sodium.................**549 mg**

Place tuna in a small bowl. Add mayonnaise and mix thoroughly. Then add lemon zest, lemon juice, carrots, celery, green onions, and celery seeds. Blend together. Serve.

LEVEL I
See previous page

LEVEL II
See previous page

LEVEL III
3 protein, 1 vegetable,
1 condiment

CHICKEN SALAD—LEVEL I

per serving:

6 oz. raw boneless, skinless chicken breast
2 Tbsp. low-fat mayonnaise
3/4 Tbsp. Dijon mustard
1/4 cup diced celery
2 Tbsp. diced green onions
1/8 tsp. black pepper
1/8 tsp. fresh dill

Calories (kcal)...........**217**
Total Fat.....................**6 g**
(26% calories from fat)
Protein ....**32 g**
Carbohydrate ....**7 g**
Cholesterol ....**79 mg**
Sodium.................**257 mg**

Poach chicken; cool and dice. Gently combine chicken with remaining ingredients and chill until ready to serve.

LEVEL I
2 protein

LEVEL II
See next page

LEVEL III
See next page

CHICKEN SALAD—LEVEL II

per serving:

8 oz. raw boneless, skinless chicken breast
2-1/2 Tbsp. low-fat mayonnaise
1 Tbsp. Dijon mustard
1/2 cup diced celery
2-1/2 Tbsp. diced green onions
1/4 tsp. black pepper
1/4 tsp. fresh dill

Calories (kcal)............**345**
Total Fat....................**12 g**
(32% calories from fat)
Protein ....**43 g**
Carbohydrate ....**14 g**
Cholesterol ....**105 mg**
Sodium.................**361 mg**

Poach chicken; cool and dice. Gently combine chicken with remaining ingredients and chill until ready to serve.

LEVEL I	LEVEL II	LEVEL III
See previous page	2-1/2 protein, 1 vegetable, 1 condiment	See below

CHICKEN SALAD—LEVEL III

per serving:

10 oz. raw boneless, skinless chicken breast
3 Tbsp. low-fat mayonnaise
1-1/2 tablespoon Dijon mustard
3/4 cup diced celery
1/3 cup diced green onions
1/2 tsp. black pepper
1/2 tsp. fresh dill

Calories (kcal)............**485**
Total Fat....................**16 g**
(26% calories from fat)
Protein ....**59 g**
Carbohydrate ....**26 g**
Cholesterol ....**132 mg**
Sodium.................**544 mg**

Poach chicken; cool and dice. Gently combine chicken with remaining ingredients and chill until ready to serve.

LEVEL I	LEVEL II	LEVEL III
See previous page	See above	3-1/2 protein, 2 vegetables, 1 condiment

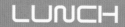

ISLAND PORK TENDERLOIN

per serving:

(See below)

16 oz. lean pork tenderloin
1/2 tsp. salt
1/4 tsp. pepper
1/2 tsp. chili powder
1/2 tsp. ground cumin
1/2 tsp. cinnamon
2 tsp. olive oil
1/4 cup brown sugar, firmly packed
1/2 Tbsp. finely chopped fresh garlic
1/2 Tbsp. Tabasco sauce

Serves 4

1. Preheat oven to 350° F.
2. Stir together salt, pepper, chili powder, cumin, and cinnamon, then coat pork with spice rub.
3. Heat oil in a 12-inch nonstick skillet over moderately high heat and brown pork, turning to brown all sides, about 4 minutes.
4. Stir together brown sugar, garlic, and Tabasco and pat onto top of tenderloin. Place pork in a roasting pan and cook in the oven for 45 minutes, or until meat thermometer inserted in center registers 160 to 165° F.
5. Slice thinly and add to Island Pork Tenderloin Salad (below and on page 50).

ISLAND PORK TENDERLOIN SALAD—LEVEL I

per serving:

1/2 orange
1 cup fresh spinach
1/2 red bell pepper, cut lengthwise into thin strips
1 Tbsp. golden raisins
1 cup shredded Napa cabbage
6 oz. Island Pork Tenderloin (see recipe above)
2 Tbsp. Cumin Vinaigrette (see recipe in Dressings)

Calories (kcal)	**556**
Total Fat	**13 g**
(37% calories from fat)	
Protein	**39 g**
Carbohydrate	**51 g**
Cholesterol	**111 mg**
Sodium	**781 mg**

1. Peel and cut orange crosswise into 1/4-inch thick slices and set aside.
2. Toss spinach, cabbage, bell pepper, and raisins in a large bowl.
3. Mound salad mixture on a large plate. Arrange pork and orange slices on top and drizzle with dressing.

LEVEL I	LEVEL II	LEVEL III
2 protein, 1/2 fruit, 2 vegetables, 3 condiments	See next page	See next page

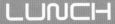

ISLAND PORK TENDERLOIN SALAD—LEVEL II

per serving:

3/4 orange

    1-1/2 cup fresh spinach

        3/4 red bell pepper, cut lengthwise into thin strips

            2 Tbsp. golden raisins

                1-1/2 cup shredded Napa cabbage

                    8 oz. Island Pork Tenderloin (see recipe on page 49)

                        3 Tbsp. Cumin Vinaigrette (see recipe in Dressings)

Calories (kcal)	**882**
Total Fat	**17 g**
(35% calories from fat)	
Protein	**52 g**
Carbohydrate	**93 g**
Cholesterol	**147 mg**
Sodium	**862 mg**

1. Peel and cut orange crosswise into 1/4-inch thick slices and set aside.
2. Toss spinach, cabbage, bell pepper, and raisins in a large bowl.
3. Mound salad mixture on a large plate. Arrange pork and orange slices on top and drizzle with dressing.

LEVEL I	LEVEL II	LEVEL III
See previous page	3 protein, 1 fruit, 3 vegetables, 4 condiments	See below

ISLAND PORK TENDERLOIN SALAD—LEVEL III

per serving:

1 orange

    2 cup fresh spinach

        1 red bell pepper, cut lengthwise into thin strips

            1/4 cup golden raisins

                2 cups shredded Napa cabbage

                    10 oz. Island Pork Tenderloin (see recipe on page 49)

                        4 Tbsp. Cumin Vinaigrette (see recipe in Dressings)

Calories (kcal)	**1,029**
Total Fat	**19 g**
(31% calories from fat)	
Protein	**69 g**
Carbohydrate	**87 g**
Cholesterol	**147 mg**
Sodium	**986 mg**

1. Peel and cut orange crosswise into 1/4-inch thick slices and set aside.
2. Toss spinach, cabbage, bell pepper, and raisins in a large bowl.
3. Mound salad mixture on a large plate. Arrange pork and orange slices on top and drizzle with dressing.

LEVEL I	LEVEL II	LEVEL III
See previous page	See above	4 protein, 2 fruits, 4 vegetables, 4 condiments

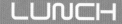
LUNCH

SHRIMP STIR-FRY—LEVEL I

per serving:

6 oz. shrimp, peeled
1/4 Tbsp. low-sodium soy sauce
1/2 tsp. rice vinegar
1/4 cup fat-free chicken or vegetable broth
1/4 tsp. minced garlic
1/4 tsp. minced ginger
1/2 cup red onion, cut in wedges
1/2 cup broccoli florets
1-1/4 cups trimmed snow peas
1-1/2 cups halved mushrooms
1/4 cup diced yellow bell pepper
1/4 cup canned water chestnuts, drained

Calories (kcal)	**332**
Total Fat	**4 g**
(9% calories from fat)	
Protein	**44 g**
Carbohydrate	**33 g**
Cholesterol	**259 mg**
Sodium	**552 mg**

1. Rinse shrimp and drain well.
2. Heat soy sauce, rice vinegar, and 2 tablespoons of chicken broth in a sauté pan over medium heat. Add garlic and ginger and sauté until tender.
3. Add all vegetables to pan and continue to sauté, stirring and adding more broth as necessary.
4. Add shrimp when vegetables are halfway cooked, and sauté until vegetables are tender and shrimp are opaque.

LEVEL I	LEVEL II	LEVEL III
2 protein, 3 vegetables	See below	See next page

SHRIMP STIR-FRY—LEVEL II

per serving:

8 oz. shrimp, peeled
1/2 Tbsp. low-sodium soy sauce
3/4 tsp. rice vinegar
1/2 cup fat-free chicken or vegetable broth
1/2 tsp. minced garlic
1/2 tsp. minced ginger
3/4 cup red onion, cut in wedges
3/4 cup broccoli florets
1-1/2 cups trimmed snow peas
1-3/4 cups halved mushrooms
1/2 cup diced yellow bell pepper
1/2 cup canned water chestnuts, drained

Calories (kcal)	**444**
Total Fat	**5 g**
(9% calories from fat)	
Protein	**61 g**
Carbohydrate	**44 g**
Cholesterol	**345 mg**
Sodium	**920 mg**

1. Rinse shrimp and drain well.
2. Heat soy sauce, rice vinegar, and 2 tablespoons of chicken broth in a sauté pan over medium heat. Add garlic and ginger and sauté until tender.
3. Add all vegetables to pan and continue to sauté, stirring and adding more broth as necessary.
4. Add shrimp when vegetables are halfway cooked, and sauté until vegetables are tender and shrimp are opaque.

LEVEL I	LEVEL II	LEVEL III
See above	2-1/2 protein, 4 vegetables	See next page

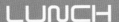

SHRIMP STIR-FRY—LEVEL III

per serving:

10 oz. shrimp, peeled
3/4 Tbsp. low-sodium soy sauce
1 tsp. rice vinegar
3/4 cup fat-free chicken or vegetable broth
3/4 tsp. minced garlic
3/4 tsp. minced ginger
1 cup red onion, cut in wedges
1-3/4 cups trimmed snow peas
1 cup broccoli florets
2 cups halved mushrooms
3/4 cup diced yellow bell pepper
3/4 cup canned water chestnuts, drained

Calories (kcal)	**571**
Total Fat	**6 g**
(9% calories from fat)	
Protein	**78 g**
Carbohydrate	**59 g**
Cholesterol	**431 mg**
Sodium	**1,290 mg**

1. Rinse shrimp and drain well.

2. Heat soy sauce, rice vinegar, and 2 tablespoons of chicken broth in a sauté pan over medium heat. Add garlic and ginger and sauté until tender.

3. Add all vegetables to pan and continue to sauté, stirring and adding more broth as necessary.

4. Add shrimp when vegetables are halfway cooked, and sauté until vegetables are tender and shrimp are opaque.

LEVEL I	LEVEL II	LEVEL III
See previous page	See previous page	3-1/2 protein, 5 vegetables

TURKEY BURGER—LEVEL I

per serving:

6 oz. extra-lean (97% fat-free) ground turkey
1-1/2 Tbsp. whole-grain bread crumbs
3 Tbsp. low-fat buttermilk
2-1/4 tsp. minced green onions
2-1/4 tsp. chopped parsley
1/4 tsp. Dijon mustard
1 dash Worcestershire sauce
Black pepper (to taste)

Calories (kcal)	**259**
Total Fat	**4.5 g**
(35% calories from fat)	
Protein	**45 g**
Carbohydrate	**13 g**
Cholesterol	**82 mg**
Sodium	**270 mg**

1. Preheat grill or broiler.

2. Combine all ingredients and form into patty.

3. Grill until cooked through (with no pink remaining), 7 to 10 minutes per side.

LEVEL I	LEVEL II	LEVEL III
2 protein, 1/2 dairy, 1 condiment	See next page	See next page

TURKEY BURGER—LEVEL II

per serving:

8 oz. extra-lean (97% fat-free) ground turkey
2 Tbsp. whole-grain bread crumbs
4 Tbsp. low-fat buttermilk
3 tsp. minced green onions
3 tsp. chopped parsley
1/2 tsp. Dijon mustard
2 dashes Worcestershire sauce
Black pepper (to taste)

Calories (kcal)............**337**
Total Fat......................**6 g**
(35% calories from fat)
Protein ....**60 g**
Carbohydrate ....**17 g**
Cholesterol ....**107 mg**
Sodium.................**351 mg**

1. Preheat grill or broiler.
2. Combine all ingredients and form into patty.
3. Grill until cooked through (with no pink remaining), 7 to 10 minutes per side.

LEVEL I
See previous page

LEVEL II
3 protein, 1/2 dairy, 1 condiment

LEVEL III
See below

TURKEY BURGER—LEVEL III

per serving:

10 oz. extra-lean (97% fat-free) ground turkey
2-1/2 Tbsp. whole-grain bread crumbs
5 Tbsp. low-fat buttermilk
3-3/4 tsp. minced green onions
3-3/4 tsp. chopped parsley
3/4 tsp. Dijon mustard
2 dashes Worcestershire sauce
Black pepper (to taste)

Calories (kcal)............**421**
Total Fat......................**8 g**
(35% calories from fat)
Protein ....**75 g**
Carbohydrate ....**21 g**
Cholesterol ....**134 mg**
Sodium.................**439 mg**

1. Preheat grill or broiler.
2. Combine all ingredients and form into patty.
3. Grill until cooked through (with no pink remaining), 7 to 10 minutes per side.

LEVEL I
See previous page

LEVEL II
See above

LEVEL III
3-1/2 protein, 1/2 dairy,
2 condiments

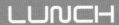

BEEF AND BROCCOLI STIR-FRY

per serving:

1/4 cup soy sauce
   1/2 red onion, sliced
      1 Tbsp. minced garlic
         1-1/2 pound top sirloin steak, sliced 1 inch thick
            1 Tbsp. sesame oil
               2 Tbsp. rice vinegar
                  1 Tbsp. minced ginger
                     4 cups broccoli florets
                        8 oz. dried soba noodles

Serves 4

Calories (kcal)............**466**	
Total Fat....................**11 g**	
(21% calories from fat)	
Protein ....**46 g**	
Carbohydrate ....**49 g**	
Cholesterol ....**99 mg**	
Sodium.............. **1,591 mg**	

1. Bring 2 quarts of water to a boil.
2. Meanwhile, heat a small amount of soy sauce in a large sauté pan, add onions and garlic, and sauté until opaque.
3. Add beef and sauté, turning often with tongs, for 7 to 10 minutes. In small bowl, stir together oil, vinegar, and ginger and add to the sauté mixture.
4. Blanch broccoli in boiling water (or microwave on high, covered and vented, for 2 minutes). Add to the meat mixture and keep warm.
5. Prepare soba noodles according to package directions. Drain, toss with the beef and broccoli, and serve.

LEVEL I	LEVEL II	LEVEL III
1-1/2 cups = 2 protein, 1 carbohydrate, 1 vegetable	2 cups = 3 protein, 1 carbohydrate, 1 vegetable	2-1/2 cups = 3 protein, 1 carbohydrate, 1 vegetable

LEMON-GARLIC CHICKEN

per serving:

1/4 cup fresh lemon juice
   2 Tbsp. molasses
      2 tsp. Worcestershire sauce
         4 garlic cloves, chopped
            2 lbs. boneless, skinless chicken thighs
               1/4 teaspoon salt
                  1/4 teaspoon black pepper
                     3 lemon wedges
                        3 parsley sprigs

Serves 3

Calories (kcal)............**153**	
Total Fat.....................**4 g**	
(24% calories from fat)	
Protein ....**21 g**	
Carbohydrate ....**8 g**	
Cholesterol ....**86 mg**	
Sodium.................**219 mg**	

1. Combine first 4 ingredients in a nonreactive dish and add chicken, turning to coat all sides. Cover and marinate in refrigerator 1 hour, turning occasionally.
2. Preheat oven to 425° F.
3. Remove chicken from dish, reserving marinade, and arrange in a shallow roasting pan coated with cooking spray. Pour reserved marinade over chicken; sprinkle with salt and pepper.
4. Bake for 20 minutes, basting occasionally with marinade. Bake without basting for 20 minutes more or until chicken is done. Serve with lemon wedges and garnish with parsley, if desired.

LEVEL I	LEVEL II	LEVEL III
6 oz. = 2 protein	8 oz. = 2-1/2 protein	10 oz. = 3 protein

DINNER

COLESLAW

per serving:

3 cups shredded green cabbage
1 cup shredded red cabbage
1 cup julienned jicama
1/2 red onion, finely chopped
2 Red Delicious apples, finely diced
1/2 cup fat-free mayonnaise
1/3 cup white vinegar
2 Tbsp. plus 2 tsp. raw sugar
2 Tbsp. plus 2 tsp. Dijon mustard
1-1/2 tsp. caraway seed
1/4 tsp. salt
1 pinch white pepper

Calories (kcal)	**38**
Total Fat	**‹1 g**
(4% calories from fat)	
Protein	**0 g**
Carbohydrate	**9 g**
Cholesterol	**0 mg**
Sodium	**171 mg**

Serves 12

1. Combine vegetables and apples in a large bowl and mix well.

2. Combine remaining ingredients in a small bowl and mix well to make dressing.

3. Pour dressing over slaw and toss until evenly coated. Cover tightly and chill before serving.

LEVEL I
1/2 cup = 1/2 vegetable

LEVEL II
1 cup = 1 vegetable

LEVEL III
2 cups = 2 vegetables

PHASE 2

ENERGY BOOSTER

The Portion Approach was designed to allow you to mix and match the foods of your choice. There are NO specific meal plans or recipes for this approach. **Just select from the Portion Approach foods listed on the following pages and eat the amounts indicated for your nutrition level.** Along with identifying the right foods to buy, the list shows you which foods fall into which categories, and the appropriate portion size to equal one serving.

For example, if you're in Phase 2 and have determined that you're at nutrition level II, you'd be allotted a specific number of servings per day from each food group, as follows:

PROTEINS	6 servings
DAIRY	2 servings
FRUITS	1 serving
VEGETABLES	3 servings
FATS	1 serving
CARBOHYDRATES	3 serving
SNACKS	2 servings

SNACKS — 2 servings (2 items from the single snack group or 1 item from the double snack group) PLUS a P90X Peak Performance Protein Bar and P90X Results and Recovery Formula drink

CONDIMENTS	1-1/2 servings

Important Note on Snacks:

There are two snack groups listed in your Portion Approach foods—the single group and the double group.

If the letters **SGL** appear beside a snack serving block on your Portion Chart, you can have any 1 item from the **single snack group**. If the letters **DBL** appear inside the snack serving block, you can have any 1 item from the **double snack group** OR any 2 items from the single snack group.

Additionally, if the words **Bar** or **Drink** appear inside a snack serving block, you can have a **P90X Peak Performance Protein Bar** and **P90X Results and Recovery Formula** drink IN ADDITION TO your allotted snack servings.

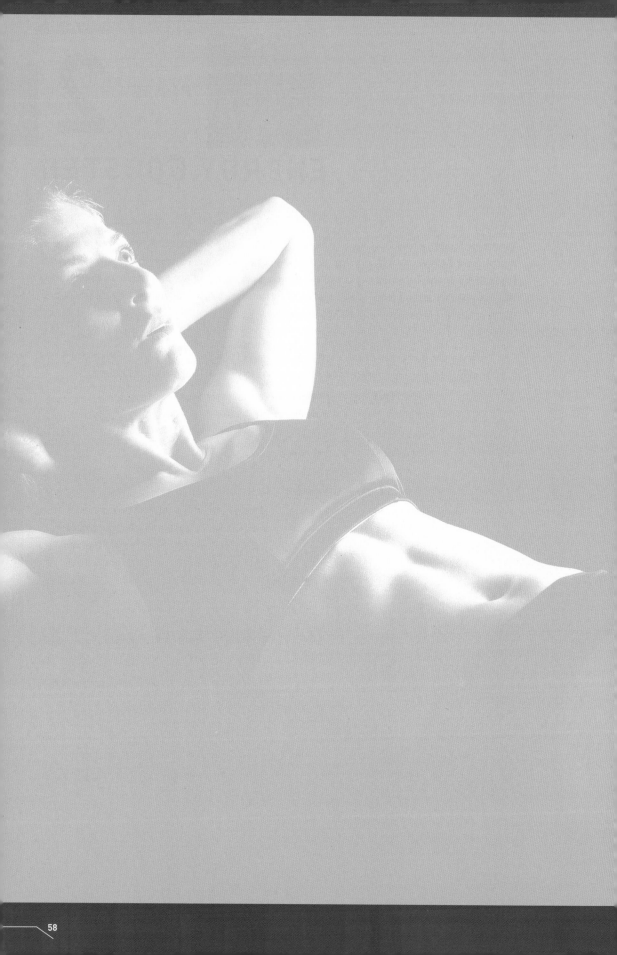

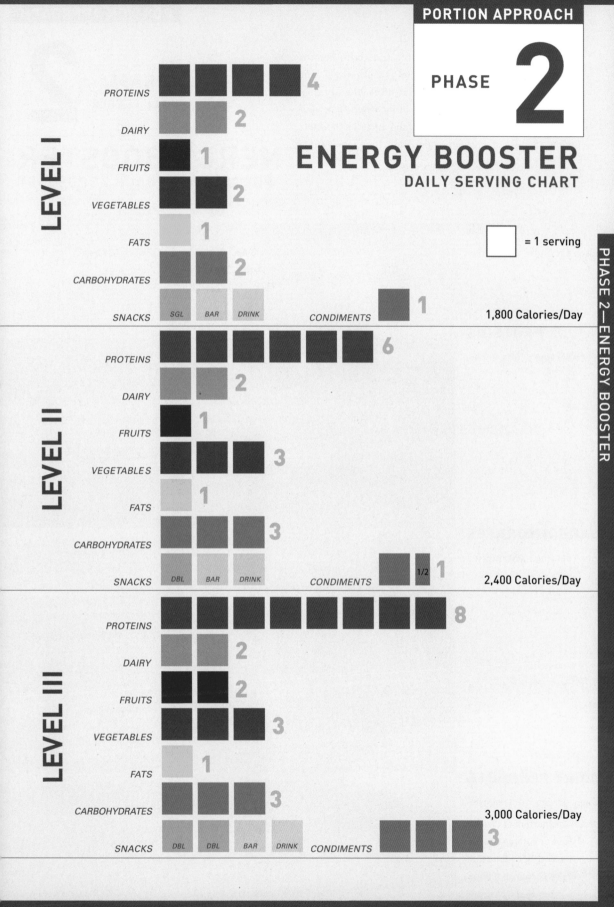

ENERGY BOOSTER
DAILY SERVING CHART

☐ = 1 serving

LEVEL I

- PROTEINS — 4
- DAIRY — 2
- FRUITS — 1
- VEGETABLES — 2
- FATS — 1
- CARBOHYDRATES — 2
- SNACKS — SGL / BAR / DRINK
- CONDIMENTS — 1

1,800 Calories/Day

LEVEL II

- PROTEINS — 6
- DAIRY — 2
- FRUITS — 1
- VEGETABLES — 3
- FATS — 1
- CARBOHYDRATES — 3
- SNACKS — DBL / BAR / DRINK
- CONDIMENTS — 1/2 1

2,400 Calories/Day

LEVEL III

- PROTEINS — 8
- DAIRY — 2
- FRUITS — 2
- VEGETABLES — 3
- FATS — 1
- CARBOHYDRATES — 3
- SNACKS — DBL / DBL / BAR / DRINK
- CONDIMENTS — 3

3,000 Calories/Day

During Phase 2, use the following list to determine which foods to purchase from the grocery store, and what amount of these foods constitutes one serving. Remember, the foods you choose to incorporate in your diet are up to you—just make sure the portions fit within the parameters of your determined nutrition level.

ENERGY BOOSTER
PORTION APPROACH FOODS LIST

FATS

Each serving = 120 calories

3 oz._Avocado	Olive oil_**1Tbsp.**
1 Tbsp._Canola oil	Olives_**4 oz.**
1Tbsp._Flaxseed oil	

PROTEINS

Each serving = 100 calories

3 oz._Boneless, skinless, chicken or turkey breast	Soy burger_**1**
6_Egg whites	Soy cheese slices_**5**
3 oz._Fish and shellfish	Tofu_**3 oz.**
3 oz._Ham slices, fat-free	Tuna_**3 oz.**
3 oz._Pork tenderloin	Turkey bacon_**2 slices**
1/3 cup_Protein powder	Veggie burger_**1**
3 oz._Red meat (top sirloin, flank steak)	Veggie dog_**1**
3 oz._Red meat, lean	

CARBOHYDRATES   GRAINS   LEGUMES   POTATOES

Each serving = 200 calories

1 medium_Bagel, whole wheat	Pancakes (3.6 oz.)_**3**
1 cup_Baked beans	Pasta or noodles_**1 cup**
1 cup_Beans (kidney, black, etc.)	Pita, whole wheat_**1 large**
1_Bran muffin (2.5 oz)	Potato_**1 medium**
2 slices_Bread (whole wheat, rye, or pumpernickel)	Quinoa_**1 cup**
1 cup_Cereal, whole grain	Refried beans, low-fat_**1 cup**
1 cup_Couscous	Rice, brown or wild_**1 cup**
12_Crackers	Sweet potato_**1 medium**
2_English muffin halves, whole wheat	Tortillas, corn_**3**
1 cup_Hummus	Tortilla, whole wheat_**1 large**
1 cup_Lentils	Waffles, whole wheat_**2**
1 cup_Oatmeal	Wheat berries_**1 cup**

DAIRY PRODUCTS

Each serving = 120 calories

Note: One portion of low-fat cheese or cottage cheese counts as either a snack or a dairy portion, not both.

1 oz._Cheese, low-fat	Parmesan cheese_**1 oz.**
1 cup_Cottage cheese, 1%	Skim milk_**8 oz.**
1 oz._Feta cheese	Soy cheese_**1 oz.**
1 oz._Goat cheese, semisoft	Soy milk_**8 oz.**
1-1/2 oz._Mozzarella, part-skim	Yogurt, plain nonfat_**8 oz.**

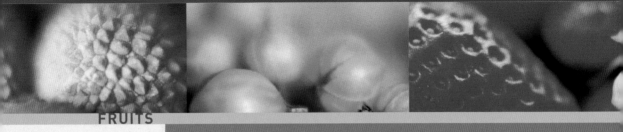

FRUITS

Each serving = 100 calories

1 medium_Apple	Nectarine_1 medium
1 cup_Apricots	Orange_1 large
1 medium_Banana	Papaya_1/2 medium
1/4 medium_Cantaloupe	Peach_1 medium
1 cup_Cherries	Pear_1 medium
1 oz._Dried fruit	Raspberries, blueberries, blackberries_1 cup
1 medium_Grapefruit	Strawberries, sliced_2 cups
1 cup_Grapes	Tangerine _1 medium
1 cup_Kiwi	Watermelon_1 cup
1/2 medium_Mango	

VEGETABLES

Each serving = 50 calories

1 serving = 1 cup
cooked vegetables,
vegetable juice,
or vegetable soup

1 serving = 2 cups
leafy greens

Asparagus	Kale
Beets	Lettuce
Bok choy	Marinara sauce
Broccoli	Mushrooms
Brussels sprouts	Peas
Cabbage	Peppers
Carrots	Spinach
Cauliflower	Sprouts
Celery	Squash (summer or winter)
Collard greens	String beans
Cucumber	Tomatoes
Eggplant	Vegetable soup

CONDIMENTS

Each serving = 50 calories
(2 Tbsp.)

BBQ and other low-fat sauces and marinades, fat-free dressings, mustard, honey, pure fruit jams

SNACKS

Single serving = 100 calories

Double serving = 200 cal.ories

Note: One portion of low-fat cheese or cottage cheese counts as either a snack or a dairy portion, not both.

Single	Double
8 oz._Cottage cheese, 1%	Cheese, low-fat_1 oz. with crackers_6
1 oz._Dried fruit	Cottage cheese, 1%_12 oz.
1/2_P90X Peak Performance Protein Bar	Hummus_4 Tbsp. with carrot sticks
1 Tbsp._Peanut butter with celery sticks	Nuts_1 oz. (almonds, cashews, pecans,
3 cups_Popcorn, light	30 pistachios)
1 large_Pretzel, sourdough	P90X Peak Performance Protein Bar_1
2 oz._Soy nuts	P90X Results and Recovery Formula_12 to 16 oz.
1-1/2 oz._String cheese	Soy nuts_4 oz.
1 oz._Turkey jerky	String cheese_3 oz.
8 oz._Yogurt, plain nonfat	Turkey jerky_2 oz.
2/3 scoop_Shakeology*	Yogurt, nonfat fruit-flavored_8 oz.

*For more information on Shakeology, please refer to page 15.

SHAKEOLOGY

Single
2/3_serving for amount

PORTION APPROACH

PHASE 2

ENERGY BOOSTER

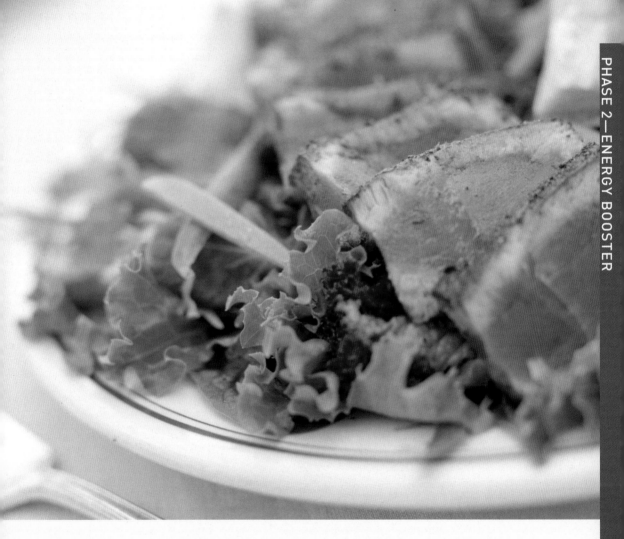

GENERAL GUIDELINES

Get the best of both worlds during Phase 2 of your training. To supply your body with additional energy for midstream performance, these recipes provide a balanced mix of carbohydrates and proteins. Mouthwatering muffins, meat loaf, and filet mignon are just a few of the appetizing dishes you'll find. There are also a variety of salads to keep it light at lunchtime.

ENERGY BOOSTER

_Recipe included

	BREAKFAST	SNACK	LUNCH	SNACK	DINNER
DAY 1	1 cup_Oatmeal 8 oz._Skim milk 1 Tbsp._Beachbody Whey Protein Powder 1/2 oz._Raisins	1_P90X Peak Performance Protein Bar 1_Results and Recovery Formula drink**	1_Shrimp Pasta Pomodoro	8 oz._Cottage cheese, 1%	6 oz._Extra-lean burger pa' 1-1/2 oz._Low-fat melted cheese 2 cups_Salad greens w/ cucumber and toma' 2 Tbsp._Dressing (your cho 1/2 cup_Fresh berries
DAY 2	1_Whole wheat bagel 8 oz._Cottage cheese, 1% 1_Orange, medium	1_P90X Peak Performance Protein Bar 1_Results and Recovery Formula drink**	1_Grilled Chicken Burrito	1 oz._Turkey jerky	6 oz._Halibut 2 Tbsp._Sauce (your choic 1_Artichoke, medium
DAY 3	1_Pear and Granola Muffin 8 oz._Nonfat yogurt 1 cup_Strawberries, sliced	1_P90X Peak Performance Protein Bar 1_Results and Recovery Formula drink**	Tuna Roll-Up: 6 oz._Tuna Salad (see Phase 1 recipes) 1_Whole wheat tortilla 1/4 cup_Sprouts and diced tomatoes	8 oz._Cottage cheese, 1%	6 oz._Chicken breast 2 Tbsp._Sauce (your choic 2 cups_Mushroom, zucchi and onion sauté 2 Tbsp._Grated Parmesan cheese
DAY 4	1_Shakeology P90X-tra Shake* 1_Banana	1_P90X Peak Performance Protein Bar 1_Results and Recovery Formula drink**	Turkey Breast Sandwich: 6 oz._Fat-free turkey breast 2 slices_Whole wheat toast 1 leaf_Lettuce 2 slices_Tomato	8 oz._Nonfat plain yogurt	6 oz._Salmon 2 Tbsp._Green Apple Sals. 1 cup_Asparagus 2 cups_Salad greens 2 Tbsp._Dressing (your cho
DAY 5	2_Whole wheat waffles 1/2_Banana, medium 2 Tbsp._Low sugar maple syrup 8 oz._Skim milk	1_P90X Peak Performance Protein Bar 1_Results and Recovery Formula drink**	1_Chicken Pita	1 oz._Turkey jerky	6 oz._Grilled Ahi Tuna Salad 2 Tbsp._Lime-Soy Vinaigrette
DAY 6	6_Egg whites 1_Breakfast Potatoes 8 oz._Cottage cheese, 1% 6 oz._Freshed-squeezed juice	1_P90X Peak Performance Protein Bar 1_Results and Recovery Formula drink**	1_White Bean and Tuna Salad	1 Tbsp._Peanut butter w/ celery sticks	6 oz._Italian Meat Loaf 1 cup_Spinach and romaine salad 1-1/2 oz._Mozzarella chee cubed 2 Tbsp._Dressing (your cho
DAY 7	3_Pancakes, 3.6 oz 2 Tbsp._Low sugar maple syrup 1 cup_Blueberries 8 oz._Skim milk 1 Tbsp._Beachbody Whey Protein Powder	1_P90X Peak Performance Protein Bar 1_Results and Recovery Formula drink** **Immediately after workout.	1_Tangy Orange Chicken Spinach Salad 2 Tbsp._Tangy Orange Vinaigrette	1-1/2 oz._String cheese	6 oz._Filet mignon 2 Tbsp._Pear and Peppercorn Sauce 1 cup_Portobello mushroor

*For more information on Shakeology, please refer to page 15.

ENERGY BOOSTER

■_Recipe included

BREAKFAST	SNACK	LUNCH	SNACK	DINNER
DAY 1 **1cup**_Oatmeal **8 oz.**_Skim milk **1 Tbsp.**_Beachbody Whey Protein Powder **1/2 oz.**_Raisins	**1**_P90X Peak Performance Protein Bar **1**_Results and Recovery Formula drink**	**1**_Shrimp Pasta Pomodoro ■	**1 oz.**_Low-fat cheese **6**_Crackers	**9 oz.**_Extra-lean burger patty **3 oz.**_Low-fat melted cheese **1**_Baked potato, medium **3 cups**_Salad greens w/ cucumber and tomatoes **3 Tbsp.**_Dressing (your choice) **1/2 cup**_Fresh berries
DAY 2 **1**_Whole wheat bagel **8 oz.**_Cottage cheese, 1% **1**_Orange, medium	**1**_P90X Peak Performance Protein Bar **1**_Results and Recovery Formula drink**	**1**_Grilled Chicken Burrito ■ **1 cup**_Gazpacho ■ (see Phase 1 recipes)	**4 Tbsp.**_Hummus w/ carrot sticks	**9 oz.**_Halibut **3 Tbsp.**_Sauce (your choice) **1**_Artichoke, medium **1 cup**_Wheat berries
DAY 3 **1**_Pear and Granola Muffin ■ **8 oz.**_Nonfat yogurt **1 cup**_Strawberries, sliced	**1**_P90X Peak Performance Protein Bar **1**_Results and Recovery Formula drink**	Tuna Roll-Up: **9 oz.**_Tuna Salad ■ (see Phase 1 recipes) **1**_Whole wheat tortilla **1/4 cup**_Sprouts and diced tomatoes	**3 cups**_Light popcorn **1-1/2 oz.**_String cheese	**9 oz.**_Chicken breast **3 Tbsp.**_Sauce (your choice) **2 cups**_Mushroom, zucchini, and onion sauté **3 Tbsp.**_Grated Parmesan cheese **1 cup**_Brown rice
DAY 4 **1**_Shakeology P90X-tra Shake* ■ **1**_Banana	**1**_P90X Peak Performance Protein Bar **1**_Results and Recovery Formula drink**	**1 cup**_Vegetable Soup ■ (see Phase 1 recipes) Turkey Breast Sandwich: **9 oz.**_Fat-free turkey breast **2 slices**_Whole wheat toast **1 leaf**_Lettuce **2 slices**_Tomato	**8 oz.**_Nonfat fuit-flavored yogurt	**9 oz.**_Salmon **3 Tbsp.**_Green Apple Salsa ■ **1 cup**_Asparagus **1**_Baked potato, medium **3 cups**_Salad greens **3 Tbsp.**_Dressing (your choice)
DAY 5 **2**_Whole wheat waffles **1/2**_Banana, medium **3 Tbsp.**_Low-sugar maple syrup **8 oz.**_Skim milk	**1**_P90X Peak Performance Protein Bar **1**_Results and Recovery Formula drink**	**1**_Chicken Pita ■	**1 oz.**_Turkey jerky **1**_Sourdough pretzel	**9 oz.**_Grilled Ahi Tuna Salad ■ **3 Tbsp.**_Lime-Soy Vinaigrette ■ **1**_Whole grain roll
DAY 6 **6**_Egg whites **1**_Breakfast Potatoes ■ **8 oz.**_Cottage cheese, 1% **6 oz.**_Freshed-squeezed juice	**1**_P90X Peak Performance Protein Bar **1**_Results and Recovery Formula drink**	**1**_White Bean and Tuna Salad ■	**1 Tbsp.**_Peanut butter w/ celery sticks **1 oz.**_Dried fruit	**9 oz.**_Italian Meat Loaf ■ **1**_Baked potato, medium **3 cups**_Spinach and romaine salad **3 oz.**_Mozzarella cheese, cubed **3 Tbsp.**_Dressing (your choice)
DAY 7 **3**_Pancakes, 3.6 oz **3 Tbsp.**_Low-sugar maple syrup **1 cup**_Blueberries **8 oz.**_Skim milk **1 Tbsp.**_Beachbody Whey Protein Powder	**1**_P90X Peak Performance Protein Bar **1**_Results and Recovery Formula drink** **Immediately after workout	**1**_Tangy Orange Chicken Spinach Salad ■ **3 Tbsp.**_Tangy Orange Vinaigrette ■	**2 oz.**_Soy nuts **3 cups**_Light popcorn	**9 oz.**_Filet mignon **3 Tbsp.**_Pear and Peppercorn Sauce ■ **1 cup**_Portobello mushrooms **1 cup**_Wild rice

*For more information on Shakeology, please refer to page 15.

PHASE 2—ENERGY BOOSTER

ENERGY BOOSTER

_Recipe included

	BREAKFAST	SNACK	LUNCH	SNACK	DINNER
DAY 1	1cup_Oatmeal 8 oz._Skim milk 1 Tbsp._Beachbody Whey Protein Powder 1/2 oz._Raisins	1_P90X Peak Performance Protein Bar 1_Results and Recovery Formula drink**	1_Shrimp Pasta Pomodoro 1 cup_Melon	1 oz._Low-fat cheese 6_Crackers 1_Sourdough pretzel	12 oz._Extra-lean burger pa 3 oz._Low-fat melted chee 1_Baked potato, medium 4 cups_Salad greens w/ cucumber and tomat 4 Tbsp._Dressing (your cho 1/2 cup_Fresh berries
DAY 2	1_Whole wheat bagel 8 oz._Cottage cheese, 1% 1_Orange, medium	1_P90X Peak Performance Protein Bar 1_Results and Recovery Formula drink**	1_Grilled Chicken Burrito 1 cup_Gazpacho (see Phase 1 recipes)	4 Tbsp._Hummus w/ carrot sticks 1 oz._Turkey jerky	12 oz._Halibut 4 Tbsp._Sauce (your choic 1_Artichoke, medium 1 cup_Wheat berries 1_Nectarine, medium
DAY 3	1_Pear and Granola Muffin 8 oz._Nonfat yogurt 1 cup_Strawberries, sliced	1_P90X Peak Performance Protein Bar 1_Results and Recovery Formula drink**	Tuna Roll-Up: 12 oz._Tuna Salad (see Phase 1 recipes) 1_Whole wheat tortilla 1/4 cup_Sprouts and diced tomatoes 1_Peach, medium	1 oz._Almonds 3 cups_Light popcorn	12 oz._Chicken breast 4 Tbsp._Sauce (your choic 2 cups_Mushroom, zucchin and onion sauté 4 Tbsp._Grated Parmesan cheese 1 cup_Brown rice
DAY 4	1_Shakeology P90X-tra Shake* 1_Banana	1_P90X Peak Performance Protein Bar 1_Results and Recovery Formula drink**	1 cup_Vegetable Soup (see Phase 1 recipes) Turkey Breast Sandwich: 12 oz._Fat-free turkey breast 2 slices_Whole wheat toast 1 leaf_Lettuce 2 slices_Tomato	8 oz._Nonfat fuit-flavored yogurt 3 cups_Light popcorn	12 oz._Salmon 4 Tbsp._Green Apple Salsa 1 cup_Asparagus 1_Baked potato, medium 4 cups_Salad greens 4 Tbsp._Dressing (your cho
DAY 5	2_Whole wheat waffles 1/2_Banana, medium 4 Tbsp._Low-sugar maple syrup 8 oz._Skim milk	1_P90X Peak Performance Protein Bar 1_Results and Recovery Formula drink**	1_Chicken Pita 1 cup_Grapes	2 oz._Soy nuts 2 oz._Turkey jerky	12 oz._Grilled Ahi Tuna Salad 4 Tbsp._Lime-Soy Vinaigrette 1_Whole grain roll
DAY 6	6_Egg whites 1_Breakfast Potatoes 8 oz._Cottage cheese, 1% 6 oz._Freshed-squeezed juice	1_P90X Peak Performance Protein Bar 1_Results and Recovery Formula drink**	1_White Bean and Tuna Salad 	8 oz._Nonfat fuit-flavored yogurt 1 Tbsp._Peanut butter w/ celery sticks	12 oz._Italian Meat Loaf 1_Baked potato, medium 4 cups_Spinach and romaine salad 3 oz._Mozzarella cheese, cubed 4 Tbsp._Dressing (your choic
DAY 7	3_Pancakes, 3.6 oz 4 Tbsp._Low-sugar maple syrup 1 cup_Blueberries 8 oz._Skim milk 1 Tbsp._Beachbody Whey Protein Powder	1_P90X Peak Performance Protein Bar 1_Results and Recovery Formula drink** **Immediately after workout.	1_Tangy Orange Chicken Spinach Salad 4 Tbsp._Tangy Orange Vinaigrette 1 cup_Strawberries, sliced	1 oz._Low-fat cheese 6_Crackers 1_Sourdough pretzel	12 oz._Filet mignon 4 Tbsp._Pear and Peppercorn Sauce 1 cup_Portobello mushroom 1 cup_Wild rice

*For more information on Shakeology, please refer to page 15.

PHASE 2

ENERGY BOOSTER

Balanced in carbohydrates and protein, but still low in fat, these recipes, including delicious sandwiches, salads, and pasta dishes, will contribute to a well-rounded long-term eating plan. They'll give you the resources you need to boost your energy and help you maintain the changes you made in Phase 1, and help you realize your potential in Phase 2.

GENERAL GUIDELINES

NOTE: All per-serving nutritional information is based on one LEVEL I serving.
LEVEL II and LEVEL III will vary, depending on portion size.

RECIPES

TANGY ORANGE VINAIGRETTE

per serving:

8 Tbsp. orange juice

4 Tbsp. red wine vinegar

2 Tbsp. olive oil

4 small cloves garlic, minced

2 oz. low-fat Parmesan cheese, grated

Calories (kcal)	**118**
Total Fat	**10 g**
(73% calories from fat)	
Protein	**4 g**
Carbohydrate	**4 g**
Cholesterol	**12 mg**
Sodium	**216 mg**

Serves 4

Combine all dressing ingredients in a small bowl and whisk.
See Tangy Orange Chicken Spinach Salad recipe.

LEVEL I	LEVEL II	LEVEL III
4 Tbsp. = 1/2 fat, 1 condiment	5 Tbsp. = 1/2 fat, 2 condiments	6 Tbsp. = 1 fat, 2 condiments

LIME-SOY VINAIGRETTE

per serving:

1/2 cup rice vinegar

1/4 cup low-sodium soy sauce

1/4 cup fresh lime juice

2 tsp. dark sesame oil

1 tsp. lemon zest

1 tsp. minced fresh ginger

2 cloves minced garlic

Calories (kcal)	**20**
Total Fat	**1 g**
(44% calories from fat)	
Protein	**1 g**
Carbohydrate	**3 g**
Cholesterol	**0 mg**
Sodium	**300 mg**

Serves 8

Combine all ingredients in a blender or food processor and process until smooth.

LEVEL I	LEVEL II	LEVEL III
4 Tbsp. = 1 condiment	3 Tbsp. = 1-1/2 condiments	4 Tbsp. = 2 condiments

GREEN APPLE SALSA

3 plum tomatoes, chopped
1 cup Granny Smith apples, cored and chopped
1/2 cup cucumber, chopped
1/2 cup corn kernels, chopped
1/2 cup red bell pepper, chopped
1/4 cup chopped green onions
1/4 cup chopped red onion
2-1/2 Tbsp. chopped fresh cilantro
1-1/2 Tbsp. fresh lime juice
1 Tbsp. seeded and chopped jalapeño
1 Tbsp. balsamic vinegar
1-1/2 tsp. sugar
3/4 tsp. salt
1/2 tsp. ground black pepper

Calories (kcal).............**24**
Total Fat....................**<1 g**
(4% calories from fat)
Protein ....**1 g**
Carbohydrate ....**6 g**
Cholesterol ....**0 mg**
Sodium ....**163 mg**

Serves 16

Combine all ingredients in a bowl, stirring well. Serve at room temperature or chilled.

LEVEL I	LEVEL II	LEVEL III
2 Tbsp. = 1 condiment	3 Tbsp. = 1-1/2 condiments	4 Tbsp. = 2 condiments

PEAR AND PEPPERCORN SAUCE

1 cup orange juice
1 Tbsp. flour
2 medium pears
1 Tbsp. Dijon mustard
1 tsp. crushed peppercorns
1/4 tsp. ground nutmeg

Calories (kcal)..............**46**
Total Fat....................**<1 g**
(6% calories from fat)
Protein ....**1 g**
Carbohydrate ....**11 g**
Cholesterol ....**0 mg**
Sodium ....**24 mg**

Serves 8

1. In a small saucepan, blend orange juice and flour and bring to a boil. Simmer until reduced to 3/4 cup.

2. Add pears, mustard, peppercorns, and nutmeg and continue cooking for several minutes, stirring until blended and thickened.

LEVEL I	LEVEL II	LEVEL III
2 Tbsp. = 1 condiment	3 Tbsp. = 1-1/2 condiments	4 Tbsp. = 2 condiments

PHASE 2—ENERGY BOOSTER

3/4 cup canned pear nectar
2 egg whites
2 Tbsp. vegetable oil
1 Tbsp. lemon juice
1 tsp. grated lemon peel
1 cup whole wheat flour
1 cup all-purpose flour
2/3 cup firmly packed brown sugar
1/2 cup low-fat granola
1 Tbsp. baking powder
1/2 tsp. ground nutmeg
1/2 tsp. salt
1-1/4 cups cored, chopped pear

Calories (kcal)	**227**
Total Fat	**5 g**
(19% calories from fat)	
Protein	**5 g**
Carbohydrate	**43 g**
Cholesterol	**0 mg**
Sodium	**284 mg**

Serves 10

1. Preheat oven to 350° F. Prepare 10 muffin cups by greasing and flouring or lining with paper liners.
2. Whisk together first five ingredients in large bowl to blend.
3. In separate medium bowl, stir both flours and sugar until no sugar lumps remain. Mix in granola, baking powder, nutmeg, and salt. Add pear; toss to coat.
4. Stir flour mixture into egg mixture until blended (batter will be thick). Divide among muffin cups.
5. Bake until golden brown and tester inserted into center comes out clean (about 20 minutes). Transfer muffins to rack and cool.

LEVEL I	LEVEL II	LEVEL III
1 muffin = 1 carbohydrate	1 muffin = 1 carbohydrate	1 muffin = 1 carbohydrate

BREAKFAST POTATOES

per serving:

1 tsp. olive oil
1 medium potato, peeled and cut into 1/2-inch cubes
2 mushrooms, chopped
1 Tbsp. chopped onion
1/4 tsp. garlic salt

Calories (kcal)	**150**
Total Fat	**5 g**
(27% calories from fat)	
Protein	**3 g**
Carbohydrate	**25 g**
Cholesterol	**0 mg**
Sodium	**522 mg**

1. Heat oil in medium nonstick skillet over medium heat. Add potatoes and cover. Cook 8 to 10 minutes or until tender, stirring occasionally.
2. Add remaining ingredients; mix lightly. Cook and stir 5 minutes or until potatoes are lightly browned and mixture is heated through.

LEVEL I	LEVEL II	LEVEL III
1 carbohydrate	1 carbohydrate	1 carbohydrate, 1/2 vegetable, 1 fat

CHICKEN PITA—LEVEL I

per serving:

6 oz. boneless, skinless chicken breast
1 whole wheat pita
1-1/2 oz. low-fat feta cheese, crumbled
1/4 cup chopped tomato
2 Tbsp. chopped red onion
1/4 cup peeled, chopped cucumber
1 squeeze fresh lemon juice

Calories (kcal)	**490**
Total Fat	**13 g**
(23% calories from fat)	
Protein	**52 g**
Carbohydrate	**41 g**
Cholesterol	**137 mg**
Sodium	**931 mg**

1. Grill chicken breast or bake in glass baking dish at 350° F for approximately 20 minutes.
2. Cool chicken and cut into 1-inch cubes.
3. Place chicken in pita and add all other ingredients. Squeeze lemon over top.

LEVEL I	LEVEL II	LEVEL III
2 protein, 1 carbohydrate, 1 dairy	See below	See next page

CHICKEN PITA—LEVEL II

per serving:

9 oz. boneless, skinless chicken breast
1 whole wheat pita
1-1/2 oz. low-fat feta cheese, crumbled
1/4 cup chopped tomato
2 Tbsp. chopped red onion
1/4 cup peeled, chopped cucumber
1 squeeze fresh lemon juice

Calories (kcal)	**583**
Total Fat	**14 g**
(21% calories from fat)	
Protein	**72 g**
Carbohydrate	**41 g**
Cholesterol	**186 mg**
Sodium	**986 mg**

1. Grill chicken breast or bake in glass baking dish at 350° F for approximately 20 minutes.
2. Cool chicken and cut into 1-inch cubes.
3. Place chicken in pita and add all other ingredients. Squeeze lemon over top.

LEVEL I	LEVEL II	LEVEL III
See above	3 protein, 1 carbohydrate, 1 dairy	See next page

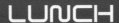

CHICKEN PITA—LEVEL III

per serving:

12 oz. boneless, skinless chicken breast

1 whole wheat pita

1-1/2 oz. low-fat feta cheese, crumbled

1/4 cup chopped tomato

2 Tbsp. chopped red onion

1/4 cup peeled, chopped cucumber

1 squeeze fresh lemon juice

Calories (kcal)............**677**
Total Fat....................**15 g**
(20% calories from fat)
Protein ....**92 g**
Carbohydrate ....**41 g**
Cholesterol ....**235 mg**
Sodium..............**1,041 mg**

1. Grill chicken breast or bake in glass baking dish at 350° F for approximately 20 minutes.
2. Cool chicken and cut into 1-inch cubes.
3. Place chicken in pita and add all other ingredients. Squeeze lemon over top.

LEVEL I	LEVEL II	LEVEL III
See previous page	See previous page	4 protein, 1 carbohydrate, 1 dairy

SHRIMP PASTA POMODORO—LEVEL I

per serving:

1 Tbsp. olive oil

1 Tbsp. chopped garlic

2 Tbsp. fat-free low-sodium chicken or vegetable broth

1/2 cup peeled and diced tomato

2 oz. whole wheat pasta

6 oz. uncooked medium shrimp

2 Tbsp. chopped basil leaves

Calories (kcal)............**150**
Total Fat......................**5 g**
(27% calories from fat)
Protein ....**3 g**
Carbohydrate ....**25 g**
Cholesterol ....**0 mg**
Sodium.................**522 mg**

1. Bring medium pot of water to boil for pasta.
2. Meanwhile, place olive oil and garlic in a large sauté pan and sauté for several minutes until lightly browned.
3. Add chicken broth and tomatoes to sauté pan; simmer for 5 to 10 minutes or until tender.
4. Cook pasta according to directions on package. Drain.
5. Add shrimp to pan and cook for several more minutes, until shrimp are opaque.
   Add basil and cooked pasta to shrimp mixture and toss.

LEVEL I	LEVEL II	LEVEL III
2 protein, 1 carbohydrate, 1 vegetable, 1/2 fat	See next page	See next page

SHRIMP PASTA POMODORO—LEVEL II

per serving:

1 Tbsp. olive oil

    1 Tbsp. chopped garlic

        2 Tbsp. fat-free low-sodium chicken or vegetable broth

            1/2 cup peeled and diced tomato

                2 oz. whole wheat pasta

                    9 oz. uncooked medium shrimp

                        2 Tbsp. chopped basil leaves

Calories (kcal)............**619**

Total Fat....................**19 g**

(27% calories from fat)

Protein ....**61 g**

Carbohydrate ....**52 g**

Cholesterol ....**388 mg**

Sodium ....**392 mg**

1. Bring medium pot of water to boil for pasta.
2. Meanwhile, place olive oil and garlic in a large sauté pan and sauté for several minutes until lightly browned.
3. Add chicken broth and tomatoes to sauté pan; simmer for 5 to 10 minutes or until tender.
4. Cook pasta according to directions on package. Drain.
5. Add shrimp to sauté pan and cook for several more minutes, until shrimp are opaque.
   Add basil and cooked pasta to shrimp mixture and toss.

LEVEL I	LEVEL II	LEVEL III
See previous page	3 protein, 1 carbohydrate, 1 vegetable, 1/2 fat	See below

SHRIMP PASTA POMODORO—LEVEL III

per serving:

1 Tbsp. olive oil

    1 Tbsp. chopped garlic

        2 Tbsp. fat-free low-sodium chicken or vegetable broth

            1/2 cup peeled and diced tomato

                2 oz. whole wheat pasta

                    12 oz. uncooked medium shrimp

                        2 Tbsp. chopped basil leaves

Calories (kcal)............**711**

Total Fat....................**20 g**

(25% calories from fat)

Protein ....**80 g**

Carbohydrate ....**53 g**

Cholesterol ....**517 mg**

Sodium ....**580 mg**

1. Bring medium pot of water to boil for pasta.
2. Meanwhile, place olive oil and garlic in a large sauté pan and sauté for several minutes until lightly browned.
3. Add chicken broth and tomatoes to sauté pan; simmer for 5 to 10 minutes or until tender.
4. Cook pasta according to directions on package. Drain.
5. Add shrimp to sauté pan and cook for several more minutes, until shrimp are opaque.
   Add basil and cooked pasta to shrimp mixture and toss.

LEVEL I	LEVEL II	LEVEL III
See previous page	See next above	3 protein, 1 carbohydrate, 1 vegetable, 1/2 fat

PHASE 2—ENERGY BOOSTER

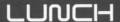

TANGY ORANGE CHICKEN SPINACH SALAD—LEVEL I   per serving:

6 oz. boneless, skinless chicken breast

2 cups spinach, stems removed

1/4 small red onion, finely sliced

1 medium tomato, diced

1/2 cup sliced mushrooms

4 Tbsp. Tangy Orange Vinaigrette (See recipe on page 68)

Calories (kcal)............**472**
Total Fat....................**16 g**
(31% calories from fat)
Protein ....**60 g**
Carbohydrate ....**20 g**
Cholesterol ....**155 mg**
Sodium.................**404 mg**

1. Cook chicken breast as desired and dice.
2. In a large bowl, combine ingredients with dressing and toss.

LEVEL I	LEVEL II	LEVEL III
2 protein, 2 vegetable, 1 fat, 1 condiment	See below	See next page

TANGY ORANGE CHICKEN SPINACH SALAD—LEVEL II   per serving:

8 oz. boneless, skinless chicken breast

3 cups spinach, stems removed

1/4 small red onion, finely sliced

1 medium tomato, diced

1 cup sliced mushrooms

5 Tbsp. Tangy Orange Vinaigrette (See recipe on page 68)

Calories (kcal)............**613**
Total Fat....................**21 g**
(31% calories from fat)
Protein ....**80 g**
Carbohydrate ....**24 g**
Cholesterol ....**206 mg**
Sodium.................**526 mg**

1. Cook chicken breast as desired and dice.
2. In a large bowl, combine ingredients with dressing and toss.

LEVEL I	LEVEL II	LEVEL III
See above	3 protein, 2 vegetable, 1 fat, 2 condiments	See next page

TANGY ORANGE CHICKEN SPINACH SALAD—LEVEL III

per serving:

10 oz. boneless, skinless chicken breast

4 cups spinach, stems removed

1/4 small red onion, finely sliced

1 medium tomato, diced

1 cup sliced mushrooms

6 Tbsp. Tangy Orange Vinaigrette (See recipe on page 68)

Calories (kcal)............**741**	
Total Fat....................**25 g**	
(31% calories from fat)	
Protein ....**99 g**	
Carbohydrate ....**26 g**	
Cholesterol ....**256 mg**	
Sodium.................**645 mg**	

1. Cook chicken breast as desired and dice.
2. In a large bowl, combine ingredients with dressing and toss.

LEVEL I	LEVEL II	LEVEL III
See previous page	See previous page	3-1/2 protein, 3 vegetable, 1 fat, 2 condiments

GRILLED CHICKEN BURRITO—LEVEL I

per serving:

6 oz. boneless, skinless chicken breast

1/2 cup chopped tomatoes

2 Tbsp. chopped cilantro

2 Tbsp. chopped red onion

1/2 cup shredded romaine lettuce

1/8 avocado

1 Tbsp. low-fat sour cream

1 small whole wheat tortilla

Calories (kcal)............**373**	
Total Fat....................**10 g**	
(23% calories from fat)	
Protein ....**44 g**	
Carbohydrate ....**27 g**	
Cholesterol ....**100 mg**	
Sodium.................**309 mg**	

1. Grill chicken breast or bake in a glass baking dish at 350° F for approximately 20 minutes. Cool and slice thinly.
2. Place tortilla in microwave between 2 paper towels and cook on high for 10 seconds.
3. Remove tortilla and pile chicken, tomatoes, cilantro, onion, lettuce, avocado, and sour cream in center. Roll into burrito.

LEVEL I	LEVEL II	LEVEL III
2 protein, 1/2 carbohydrate, 1 vegetable, 1 condiment	See next page	See next page

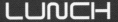

GRILLED CHICKEN BURRITO—LEVEL II

per serving:

9 oz. boneless, skinless chicken breast
1/2 cup chopped tomatoes
2 Tbsp. chopped cilantro
2 Tbsp. chopped red onion
1/2 cup shredded romaine lettuce
1/8 avocado
1 Tbsp. low-fat sour cream
1 small whole wheat tortilla

Calories (kcal)	**467**
Total Fat	**11 g**
(20% calories from fat)	
Protein	**64 g**
Carbohydrate	**27 g**
Cholesterol	**149 mg**
Sodium	**364 mg**

1. Grill chicken breast or bake in a glass baking dish at 350° F for approximately 20 minutes.
   Cool and slice thinly.
2. Place tortilla in microwave between 2 paper towels and cook on high for 10 seconds.
3. Remove tortilla and pile chicken, tomatoes, cilantro, onion, lettuce, avocado,
   and sour cream in center. Roll into burrito.

LEVEL I	LEVEL II	LEVEL III
See previous page	3 protein, 1/2 carbohydrate, 1 vegetable, 1 condiment	See below

GRILLED CHICKEN BURRITO—LEVEL III

per serving:

12 oz. boneless, skinless chicken breast
1/2 cup chopped tomatoes
2 Tbsp. chopped cilantro
2 Tbsp. chopped red onion
1/2 cup shredded romaine lettuce
1/8 avocado
1 Tbsp. low-fat sour cream
1 small whole wheat tortilla

Calories (kcal)	**555**
Total Fat	**12 g**
(19% calories from fat)	
Protein	**83 g**
Carbohydrate	**27 g**
Cholesterol	**198 mg**
Sodium	**419 mg**

1. Grill chicken breast or bake in a glass baking dish at 350° F for approximately 20 minutes.
   Cool and slice thinly.
2. Place tortilla in microwave between 2 paper towels and cook on high for 10 seconds.
3. Remove tortilla and pile chicken, tomatoes, cilantro, onion, lettuce, avocado,
   and sour cream in center. Roll into burrito.

LEVEL I	LEVEL II	LEVEL III
See previous page	See above	4 protein, 1/2 carbohydrate, 1 vegetable, 1 condiment

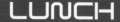

WHITE BEAN AND TUNA SALAD—LEVEL I

per serving:

6 oz. tuna canned in water, drained

1 cup cooked white beans

1/2 cup chopped green pepper

1/2 cup chopped yellow pepper

2 Tbsp. chopped green onion

2 Tbsp. chopped fresh parsley

1 dash white pepper

1 Tbsp. lemon juice

1 Tbsp. lemon zest

1 tsp. olive oil

Calories (kcal)............**540**

Total Fat.....................**7 g**

(11% calories from fat)

Protein ....**63 g**

Carbohydrate ....**58 g**

Cholesterol ....**51 mg**

Sodium.................**595 mg**

1. Place first 6 ingredients in a glass bowl and mix thoroughly.

2. In a separate bowl, mix remaining ingredients until blended and drizzle over salad.

LEVEL I	LEVEL II	LEVEL III
2 protein, 1 carbohydrate, 1 vegetable, 1 fat	See below	See next page

WHITE BEAN AND TUNA SALAD—LEVEL II

per serving:

9 oz. tuna canned in water, drained

1 cup cooked white beans

3/4 cup chopped green pepper

3/4 cup chopped yellow pepper

3 Tbsp. chopped green onion

3 Tbsp. chopped fresh parsley

1 dash white pepper

2 Tbsp. lemon juice

2 Tbsp. lemon zest

2 tsp. olive oil

Calories (kcal)............**710**

Total Fat.....................**12 g**

(19% calories from fat)

Protein ....**86 g**

Carbohydrate ....**66 g**

Cholesterol ....**77 mg**

Sodium.................**888 mg**

1. Place first 6 ingredients in a glass bowl and mix thoroughly.

2. In a separate bowl, mix remaining ingredients until blended and drizzle over salad.

LEVEL I	LEVEL II	LEVEL III
See above	3 protein, 1 carbohydrate, 2 vegetable, 1 fat	See next page

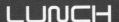

per serving:

12 oz. tuna canned in water, drained

1 cup cooked white beans

1 cup chopped green pepper

1 cup chopped yellow pepper

4 Tbsp. chopped green onion

3 Tbsp. chopped fresh parsley

1 dash white pepper

3 Tbsp. lemon juice

3 Tbsp. lemon zest

1 Tbsp. olive oil

Calories (kcal)............**936**	
Total Fat....................**18 g**	
(27% calories from fat)	
Protein ....**110 g**	
Carbohydrate ....**86 g**	
Cholesterol ....**102 mg**	
Sodium ....**1,181 mg**	

1. Place first 6 ingredients in a glass bowl and mix thoroughly.
2. In a separate bowl, mix remaining ingredients until blended and drizzle over salad.

LEVEL I
See previous page

LEVEL II
See previous page

LEVEL III
4 protein, 1 carbohydrate, 3 vegetable, 1 fat

 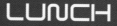

ITALIAN MEAT LOAF

per serving:

1/2 cup diced onions	
2 Tbsp. fat-free low-sodium chicken or vegetable broth	
2 Tbsp. minced garlic	
1-1/2 lbs. ground turkey breast	
1/2 cup whole-grain bread crumbs	
1/2 cup + 2 Tbsp. low-sodium, low-fat marinara sauce	
2 Tbsp. chopped fresh basil	
2 Tbsp. chopped fresh Italian parsley	

Calories (kcal)............**297**
Total Fat......................**3 g**
(8% calories from fat)
Protein ....**45 g**
Carbohydrate ....**20 g**
Cholesterol ....**106 mg**
Sodium ....**410 mg**

Serves 4

1. Preheat oven to 350° F.
2. Sauté onions in chicken broth until lightly browned; add garlic and cook 5 minutes more. Remove from heat.
3. When cool, combine in large bowl with ground turkey, bread crumbs, 1/2 cup marinara sauce, basil, and parsley. Form mixture into a loaf. Shape and place in an ungreased loaf pan.
4. Brush with 2 Tbsp. marinara sauce and bake 30 to 45 minutes, or until cooked through.
5. Drain fat and let cool 20 minutes before cutting into 8 slices.

LEVEL I	LEVEL II	LEVEL III
2 slices (6 oz.) = 2 protein, 1 vegetable	3 slices (9 oz.) = 3 protein, 1 vegetable	4 slices (12 oz.) = 4 protein, 1 vegetable

GRILLED AHI TUNA SALAD—LEVEL I

per serving:

6 oz. yellowfin tuna (ahi)	
2 cups arugula leaves	
2 Tbsp. soybeans	
1/4 cup canned water chestnuts, drained	
1/2 cup cubed papaya	
1 tsp. sesame seeds	
2 Tbsp. Lime-Soy Vinaigrette (see recipe on page 68)	

Calories (kcal)............**352**
Total Fat......................**8 g**
(20% calories from fat)
Protein ....**51 g**
Carbohydrate ....**20 g**
Cholesterol ....**77 mg**
Sodium ....**79 mg**

1. Grill tuna for 2 to 4 minutes on each side, depending on your preference for doneness.
2. Cut into thin slices.
3. Arrange arugula leaves on a large plate. Sprinkle soybeans and water chestnuts on top.
4. Add papaya and ahi last. Garnish with sesame seeds and drizzle with dressing.

LEVEL I	LEVEL II	LEVEL III
2 protein, 1/2 fruit, 2 vegetables	See next page	See next page

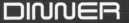

GRILLED AHI TUNA SALAD—LEVEL II

per serving:

9 oz. yellowfin tuna (ahi)

3 cups arugula leaves

2 Tbsp. soybeans

1/4 cup canned water chestnuts, drained

1/2 cup cubed papaya

1 tsp. sesame seeds

3 Tbsp. Lime-Soy Vinaigrette (see recipe on page 68)

Calories (kcal)............**449**

Total Fat.....................**9 g**

(17% calories from fat)

Protein ....**71 g**

Carbohydrate ....**21 g**

Cholesterol ....**115 mg**

Sodium.................**116 mg**

1. Grill tuna for 2 to 4 minutes on each side, depending on your preference for doneness.
2. Cut into thin slices.
3. Arrange arugula leaves on a large plate. Sprinkle soybeans and water chestnuts on top.
4. Add papaya and ahi last. Garnish with sesame seeds and drizzle with dressing.

LEVEL I	LEVEL II	LEVEL III
See previous page	2 protein, 1/2 fruit, 2 vegetables	See below

GRILLED AHI TUNA SALAD—LEVEL III

per serving:

12 oz. yellowfin tuna (ahi)

4 cups arugula leaves

2 Tbsp. soybeans

1/4 cup canned water chestnuts, drained

1/2 cup cubed papaya

1 tsp. sesame seeds

4 Tbsp. Lime-Soy Vinaigrette (see recipe on page 68)

Calories (kcal)............**546**

Total Fat.....................**10 g**

(16% calories from fat)

Protein ....**91 g**

Carbohydrate ....**22 g**

Cholesterol ....**153 mg**

Sodium.................**153 mg**

1. Grill tuna for 2 to 4 minutes on each side, depending on your preference for doneness.
2. Cut into thin slices.
3. Arrange arugula leaves on a large plate. Sprinkle soybeans and water chestnuts on top.
4. Add papaya and ahi last. Garnish with sesame seeds and drizzle with dressing.

LEVEL I	LEVEL II	LEVEL III
See previous page	See above	2 protein, 1/2 fruit, 2 vegetables

 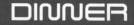

PHASE 3

ENDURANCE MAXIMIZER

The Portion Approach was designed to allow you to mix and match the foods of your choice. There are NO specific meal plans or recipes for this approach. **Just select from the Portion Approach foods listed on the following pages and eat the amounts indicated for your nutrition level.** Along with identifying the right foods to buy, the list shows you which foods fall into which categories, and the appropriate portion size to equal one serving.

For example, if you're in Phase 3 and have determined that you're at nutrition level II, you'd be allotted a specific number of servings per day from each food group, as follows:

PROTEINS	3 servings
DAIRY	1 servings
FRUITS	3 serving
VEGETABLES	3 servings
FATS	1 serving
CARBOHYDRATES	4 serving
SNACKS	3 servings
CONDIMENTS	3 servings

SNACKS — (2 items from the single snack group or 1 item from the double snack group) PLUS a P90X Peak Performance Protein Bar and P90X Results and Recovery Formula drink

Important Note on Snacks:

There are two snack groups listed in your Portion Approach foods—the single group and the double group.

If the letters **SGL** appear beside a snack serving block on your Portion Chart, you can have any 1 item from the **single snack group**. If the letters **DBL** appear inside the snack serving block, you can have any 1 item from the **double snack group** OR any 2 items from the single snack group.

Additionally, if the words **Bar** or **Drink** appear inside a snack serving block, you can have a **P90X Peak Performance Protein Bar** and **P90X Results and Recovery Formula** drink IN ADDITION TO your allotted snack servings.

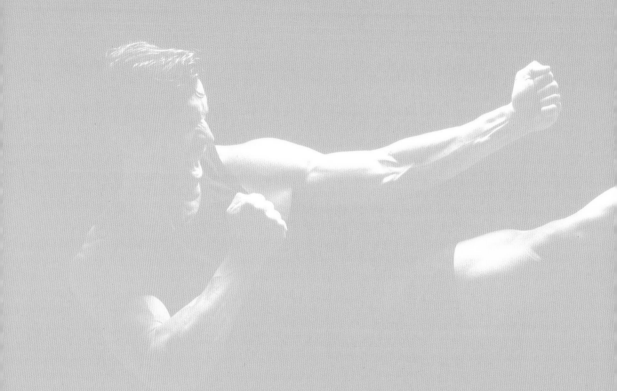

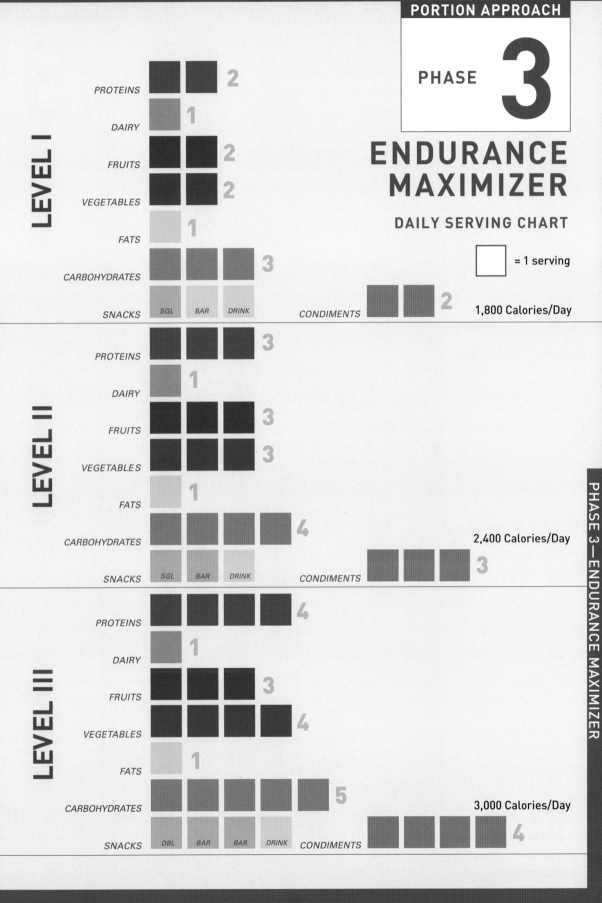

During Phase 3, use the following list to determine which foods to purchase from the grocery store, and what amount of these foods constitutes one serving. Remember, the foods you choose to incorporate in your diet are up to you— just make sure the portions fit within the parameters of your determined nutrition level.

ENDURANCE MAXIMIZER

PORTION APPROACH FOODS LIST

FATS

Each serving = 120 calories

3 oz._Avocado	Olive oil_**1Tbsp.**
1 Tbsp._Canola oil	Olives_**4 oz.**
1Tbsp._Flaxseed oil	

PROTEINS

Each serving = 100 calories

3 oz._Boneless, skinless, chicken or turkey breast	Soy burger_**1**
6_Egg whites	Soy cheese slices_**5**
3 oz._Fish and shellfish	Tofu_**3 oz.**
3 oz._Ham slices, fat-free	Tuna_**3 oz.**
3 oz._Pork tenderloin	Turkey bacon_**2 slices**
1/3 cup_Protein powder	Veggie burger_**1**
3 oz._Red meat (top sirloin, flank steak)	Veggie dog_**1**
3 oz._Red meat, lean	

CARBOHYDRATES   GRAINS   LEGUMES   POTATOES

Each serving = 200 calories

1 medium_Bagel, whole wheat	Pancakes (3.6 oz.)_**3**
1 cup_Baked beans	Pasta or noodles_**1 cup**
1 cup_Beans (kidney, black, etc.)	Pita, whole wheat_**1 large**
1_Bran muffin (2.5 oz.)	Potato_**1 medium**
2 slices_Bread (whole wheat, rye, or pumpernickel)	Quinoa_**1 cup**
1 cup_Cereal, whole grain	Refried beans, low-fat_**1 cup**
1 cup_Couscous	Rice, brown or wild_**1 cup**
12_Crackers	Sweet potato_**1 medium**
2_English muffin halves, whole wheat	Tortillas, corn_**3**
1 cup_Hummus	Tortilla, whole wheat_**1 large**
1 cup_Lentils	Waffles, whole wheat_**2**
1 cup_Oatmeal	Wheat berries_**1 cup**

DAIRY PRODUCTS

Each serving = 120 calories

Note: One portion of low-fat cheese or cottage cheese counts as either a snack or a dairy portion, not both.

1-1/2 oz._Cheese, low-fat	Parmesan cheese_**1 oz.**
1 cup_Cottage cheese, 1%	Skim milk_**8 oz.**
1-1/2 oz._Feta cheese	Soy cheese_**1-1/2 oz.**
1-1/2 oz._Goat cheese, semisoft	Soy milk_**8 oz.**
1-1/2 oz._Mozzarella, part-skim	Yogurt, plain nonfat_**8 oz.**

FRUITS

Each serving = 100 calories

1 medium_Apple	Nectarine_**1 medium**
1 cup_Apricots	Orange_**1 large**
1 medium_Banana	Papaya_**1/2 medium**
1/4 medium_Cantaloupe	Peach_**1 medium**
1 cup_Cherries	Pear_**1 medium**
1 oz._Dried fruit	Raspberries, blueberries, blackberries_**1 cup**
1 medium_Grapefruit	Strawberries, sliced_**2 cups**
1 cup_Grapes	Tangerine _**1 medium**
1 cup_Kiwi	Watermelon_**1 cup**
1/2 medium_Mango	

VEGETABLES

Each serving = 50 calories

1 serving = 1 cup
cooked vegetables,
vegetable juice,
or vegetable soup

1 serving = 2 cups
leafy greens

Asparagus	Kale
Beets	Lettuce
Bok choy	Marinara sauce
Broccoli	Mushrooms
Brussels sprouts	Peas
Cabbage	Peppers
Carrots	Spinach
Cauliflower	Sprouts
Celery	Squash (summer or winter)
Collard greens	String beans
Cucumber	Tomatoes
Eggplant	Vegetable soup

CONDIMENTS

Each serving = 50 calories
(2 Tbsp.)

BBQ and other low-fat sauces and marinades, fat-free dressings, mustard, honey, pure fruit jams

SNACKS

Single serving = 100 calories
Double serving = 200 calories

Note: One portion of low-fat cheese or cottage cheese counts as either a snack or a dairy portion, not both.

Single	Double
1 oz._Dried fruit	Bean dip_**4 Tbsp.** with chips_**1 oz.**
1 medium piece_ Fruit	Cheese, low-fat_**1 oz.** with crackers_**6**
12_Mini-rice cakes	Hummus_**4 Tbsp.** with carrot sticks
1 Tbsp._Peanut butter with celery sticks	Nuts_**1 oz.** (almonds, cashews, pecans,
1 oz._Pita chips	30 pistachios)
3 cups_Popcorn, light	P90X Peak Performance Protein Bar_**1**
1 large_Pretzel, sourdough	P90X Results and Recovery Formula_**12–16 oz.**
2 oz._Soy nuts	Soy nuts_**4 oz.**
1-1/2 oz._String cheese	String cheese_**3 oz.**
1 oz._Tortilla chips, low-fat	Yogurt, nonfat fruit-flavored_**8 oz.**
8 oz._Yogurt, plain nonfat	
2/3 scoop_Shakeology*	

*For more information on Shakeology, please refer to page 15.

SHAKEOLOGY

Single
2/3_serving for amount

PORTION APPROACH

PHASE **3**

ENDURANCE MAXIMIZER

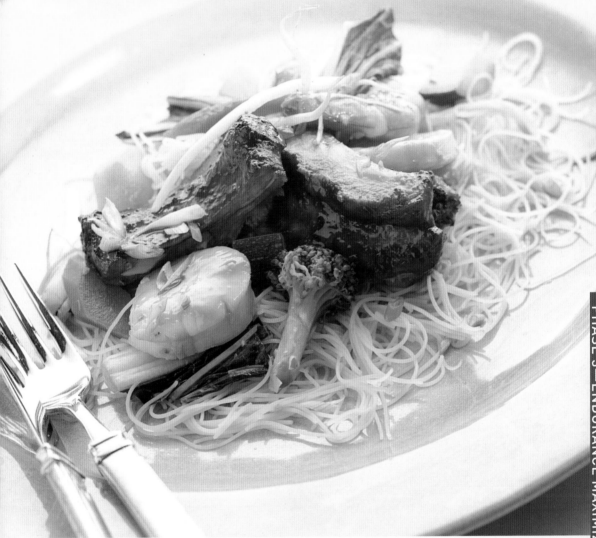

GENERAL GUIDELINES

If you've been craving those traditional carb favorites like pancakes, pasta, and potatoes, then welcome to Phase 3. The high-carbohydrate recipes in this section will help keep you energized during the final stretch. Additionally, there are plenty of great-tasting meat, poultry, and seafood entrees to ensure fast muscle recovery.

ENDURANCE MAXIMIZER

■_Recipe included

BREAKFAST	SNACK	LUNCH	SNACK	DINNER
DAY 1 **1**_Blueberry Muffin ■ **8 oz.**_Plain nonfat yogurt **1 cup**_Berries	**1**_Results and Recovery Formula drink**	**1**_Veggie burger **1/2**_Whole grain bun **2 cups**_Salad greens **2 Tbsp.**_Dressing (your choice)	**3**_Fig Newtons **1**_Sourdough pretzel	**6 oz.**_Chicken **2 Tbsp.**_Apricot Sauce ■ **1/2 cups**_Baked yam, medium **1 cup**_Green beans, steamed **1/4**_Mango
DAY 2 **2**_Whole grain waffles **1 Tbsp.**_Peanut butter **8 oz.**_Skim milk **1**_Banana, medium	**1**_Results and Recovery Formula drink**	**1**_Pasta Salad ■	**12**_Mini–rice cakes **1**_Frozen fruit bar	**6 oz.**_Halibut **2 Tbsp.**_Mustard Cream Sauce ■ **1 cup**_Brown rice **2 cups**_Spinach, steamed **1 cup**_Raspberries
DAY 3 **1**_Whole grain roll **1/2 cup**_Low-fat ricotta cheese **4 slices**_Roma tomato **2 tsp.**_Olive oil **1 cup**_Cantaloupe pieces	**1**_Results and Recovery Formula drink**	**1 cup**_Black and White Bean Chili ■ **2 cups**_Salad greens **2 Tbsp.**_Dressing (your choice)	**3 cups**_Popcorn, light **4 oz.**_Nonfat frozen yogurt	**6 oz.**_Flank steak, grilled **2 Tbsp.**_Steak sauce **1**_Baked potato, medium **1 cup**_Onion, zucchini, and stewed tomato sau■ **1**_Nectarine, medium
DAY 4 **1/2 cup**_Low-fat granola **8 oz.**_Plain nonfat yogurt **1 cup**_Strawberries, sliced	**1**_Results and Recovery Formula drink**	**1**_Stuffed Baked Potato ■ **2 cups**_Salad greens **2 Tbsp.**_Dressing (your choice)	**1 oz.**_Dried fruit **2 oz.**_Soy nuts	**6 oz.**_Mediterranean Shri■ Kebabs ■ **1 cup**_White rice **1**_Orange, medium
DAY 5 **3**_Oatmeal Pancakes ■ **2 Tbsp.**_Low sugar maple syrup **1 cup**_Applesauce	**1**_Results and Recovery Formula drink**	**1**_Grilled Veggie Focaccia ■ **1 cup**_Melon pieces	**8 oz.**_Fruit sorbet **12**_Mini–rice cakes	**6 oz.**_Chicken **2 Tbsp.**_Barbecue Sauce ■ **1 cup**_Nonfat baked beans **2 cups**_Salad greens **2 Tbsp.**_Dressing (your cho■
DAY 6 **8 oz.**_Cottage cheese, 1% **1 cup**_Pineapple chunks **2 slices**_Whole wheat toast **2 tsp.**_Pure fruit jam	**1**_Results and Recovery Formula drink**	**1**_Spicy Chinese Noodles ■	**1**_Sourdough pretzel **4 oz.**_Nonfat frozen yogurt	**6 oz.**_Salmon **2 Tbsp.**_Dijonnaise Sauce ■ **1 cup**_Quinoa **1 cup**_Broccoli, steamed **1 cup**_Grapes
DAY 7 **1**_Whole wheat bagel **2 Tbsp.**_Fat-free cream cheese **8 oz.**_Plain nonfat yogurt **1 cup**_Berries	**1**_Results and Recovery Formula drink**	**1**_Vegetarian Tostada ■	**1**_Medium piece fresh fruit **1 Tbsp.**_Peanut butter w/ celery sticks	**6 oz.**_Pork Chop with Appl■ and Sweet Potato ■ **1 cup**_Peas **2 cups**_Salad greens **2 Tbsp.**_Dressing (your cho■

**Immediately after workout.

ENDURANCE MAXIMIZER

▬_Recipe included

BREAKFAST	SNACK	LUNCH	SNACK	DINNER
↘_1 **1**_Blueberry Muffin ▬ **8 oz.**_Plain nonfat yogurt **1 cup**_Berries	**1**_Results and Recovery Formula drink**	**1**_Veggie burger **1**_Whole grain bun **3 cups**_Salad greens **3 Tbsp.**_Dressing (your choice) **1 cup**_Melon pieces	**1 oz.**_Almonds **1-1/2 oz.**_String cheese	**9 oz.**_Chicken **3 Tbsp.**_Apricot Sauce ▬ **1**_Baked yam, medium **1 cup**_Green beans, steamed **3 cups**_Salad greens **3 Tbsp.**_Dressing (your choice) **1/4**_Mango
↘_2 **3**_Whole grain waffles **2 Tbsp.**_Peanut butter **8 oz.**_Skim milk **1**_Banana, medium	**1**_Results and Recovery Formula drink**	**1**_Pasta Salad ▬ **1 cup**_Melon pieces	**1 oz.**_Low-fat tortilla chips **4 Tbsp.**_Bean dip **1**_Medium piece fresh fruit	**9 oz.**_Halibut **3 Tbsp.**_Mustard Cream Sauce ▬ **1 cup**_Brown rice **3 cups**_Spinach, steamed **1**_Peach, medium
↘_3 **1**_Whole grain roll **1/2 cup**_Low-fat ricotta cheese **4 slices**_Roma tomato **2 Tsp.**_Olive oil **1 cup**_Cantaloupe pieces	**1**_Results and Recovery Formula drink**	**2 cups**_Black and White Bean Chili ▬ **3 cups**_Salad greens **3 Tbsp.**_Dressing (your choice) **1 cup**_Grapes	**3 cups**_Popcorn, light **8 oz.**_Nonfat fruit-flavored yogurt	**9 oz.**_Flank steak, grilled **3 Tbsp.**_Steak sauce **1**_Baked potato, medium **2 cups**_Onion, zucchini, and stewed tomato sauté **1**_Nectarine, medium
↘_4 **1/2 cup**_Low-fat granola **8 oz.**_Plain nonfat yogurt **1 cup**_Strawberries, sliced	**1**_Results and Recovery Formula drink**	**2**_Stuffed Baked Potato ▬ **3 cups**_Salad greens **3 Tbsp.**_Dressing (your choice) **1**_Orange, medium	**1 oz.**_Pita chips **4 Tbsp.**_Hummus w/ carrot sticks	**9 oz.**_Mediterranean Shrimp Kebabs ▬ **1 cup**_White rice **3 cups**_Salad greens **3 Tbsp.**_Dressing (your choice) **1 cup**_Melon pieces
↘_5 **3**_Oatmeal Pancakes ▬ **3 Tbsp.**_Low sugar maple syrup **1 cup**_Applesauce **8 oz.**_Skim milk	**1**_Results and Recovery Formula drink**	**1**_Grilled Veggie Focaccia ▬ **1 cup**_Tabouli salad **1**_Peach, medium	**8 oz.**_Fruit sorbet **1-1/2 oz.**_String cheese **6**_Crackers	**9 oz.**_Chicken **3 Tbsp.**_Barbecue Sauce ▬ **1 cup**_Nonfat baked beans **3 cups**_Salad greens **3 Tbsp.**_Dressing (your choice) **1 cup**_Fruit salad
↘_6 **8 oz.**_Cottage cheese, 1% **1 cup**_Pineapple chunks **2 slices**_Whole wheat toast **3 tsp.**_Pure fruit jam	**1**_Results and Recovery Formula drink**	**1**_Spicy Chinese Noodles ▬ **3 cups**_Salad greens **3 Tbsp.**_Dressing (your choice) **1 cup**_Fruit salad	**1 oz.**_Almonds **1 oz.**_Dried fruit **8 oz.**_Nonfat plain yougurt	**9 oz.**_Salmon **3 Tbsp.**_Dijonnaise Sauce ▬ **1 cup**_Quinoa **1 cup**_Broccoli, steamed **1 cup**_Grapes
↘_7 **1**_Whole wheat bagel **2 Tbsp.**_Fat-free cream cheese **8 oz.**_Plain nonfat yogurt **1 cup**_Berries	**1**_Results and Recovery Formula drink**	**1**_Vegetarian Tostada ▬ **1 cup**_Fruit salad	**1 oz.**_Cashews **1 oz.**_Dried fruit	**9 oz.**_Pork Chop with Apple and Sweet Potato ▬ **1 cup**_Peas **3 cups**_Salad greens **3 Tbsp.**_Dressing (your choice)

**Immediately after workout.

ENDURANCE MAXIMIZER

■ _Recipe included

	BREAKFAST	SNACK	LUNCH	SNACK	DINNER
DAY 1	1_Blueberry Muffin ■ 8 oz._Plain nonfat yogurt 1 cup_Berries 1/2 cup_Low-fat granola	1_Results and Recovery Formula drink**	1_Veggie burger 1_Whole grain bun 4 cups_Salad greens 4 Tbsp._Dressing (your choice) 1 cup_Melon pieces	1 oz._Almonds 1 oz._Dried fruit 8 oz._Nonfat frozen yogurt	12 oz._Chicken 4 Tbsp._Apricot Sauce ■ 1_Baked yam, medium 1 cup_Green beans, steam 4 cups_Salad greens 4 Tbsp._Dressing (your ch◄ 1/4_Mango
DAY 2	4_Whole grain waffles 2 Tbsp._Peanut butter 8 oz._Skim milk 1_Banana, medium	1_Results and Recovery Formula drink**	1_Pasta Salad ■ 1 cup_Melon pieces	1 oz._Low-fat tortilla chips 4 Tbsp._Bean dip 1_Frozen fruit bar	12 oz._Halibut 4 Tbsp._Mustard Cream Sauce ■ 1 cup_Brown rice 3 cups_Spinach, steamed 1_Peach, medium
DAY 3	1_Whole grain roll 1/2 cup_Low-fat ricotta cheese 4 slices_Roma tomato 2 Tsp._Olive oil 1 cup_Cantaloupe pieces	1_Results and Recovery Formula drink**	2 cups_Black and White Bean Chili ■ 4 cups_Salad greens 4 Tbsp._Dressing (your choice) 1 cup_Grapes 6_Crackers	3 cups_Popcorn, light 8 oz._Nonfat fruit-flavored yogurt 2 oz._Soy nuts	12 oz._Flank steak, grille 4 Tbsp._Steak sauce 1_Baked potato, medium 2 cups_Onion, zucchini, a◄ stewed tomato sa◄ 1_Nectarine, medium
DAY 4	1 cup_Low-fat granola 8 oz._Plain nonfat yogurt 1 cup_Strawberries, sliced	1_Results and Recovery Formula drink**	2_Stuffed Baked Potato ■ 4 cups_Salad greens 4 Tbsp._Dressing (your choice) 1_Orange, medium	1 oz._Pita chips 4 Tbsp._Hummus w/ carrot sticks 1 oz._Dried fruit	12 oz._Mediterranean Shrimp Kebabs ■ 1 cup_White rice 4 cups_Salad greens 4 Tbsp._Dressing (your choice) 1 cup_Melon pieces
DAY 5	4_Oatmeal Pancakes ■ 4 Tbsp._Low-sugar maple syrup 1 cup_Applesauce 8 oz._Skim milk	1_Results and Recovery Formula drink**	1_Grilled Veggie Focaccia ■ 1 cup_Tabouli salad 1_Peach, medium	8 oz._Fruit sorbet 1-1/2 oz._String cheese 6_Crackers 3 cups_Popcorn, light	12 oz._Chicken 4 Tbsp._Barbecue Sauce ■ 1 cup_Nonfat baked beans 4 cups_Salad greens 4 Tbsp._Dressing (your choice) 1 cup_Fruit salad
DAY 6	8 oz._Cottage cheese, 1% 1 cup_Pineapple chunks 4 slices_Whole wheat toast 3 tsp._Pure fruit jam	1_Results and Recovery Formula drink**	1_Spicy Chinese Noodles ■ 4 cups_Salad greens 4 Tbsp._Dressing (your choice) 1 cup_Fruit salad	1_Sourdough pretzel 8 oz._Frozen yogurt 1_Medium piece of fruit	12 oz._Salmon 4 Tbsp._Dijonnaise Sauce ■ 1 cup_Quinoa 1 cup_Broccoli, steamed 1 cup_Grapes
DAY 7	1_Whole wheat bagel 2 Tbsp._Fat-free cream cheese 8 oz._Plain nonfat yogurt 1 cup_Berries 1/2 cup_Low-fat granola	1_Results and Recovery Formula drink**	1_Vegetarian Tostada ■ 1 cup_Fruit salad	1 oz._Cashews 1 oz._Dried fruit 1_Sourdough pretzel	12 oz._Pork Chop with Appl and Sweet Potato ■ 1 cup_Peas 4 cups_Salad greens 4 Tbsp._Dressing (your choice)

**Immediately
after workout.

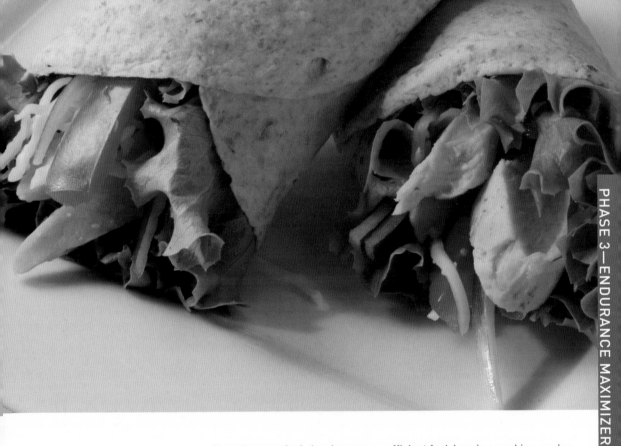

PHASE 3

ENDURANCE MAXIMIZER

Now that your body has become an efficient fuel-burning machine, you're ready for an athletic diet that'll help you push your body to the limit. These recipes, full of complex carbohydrates, lean protein, and low fat, will give you the extra push you need to maximize your endurance and get in the best shape of your life.

GENERAL GUIDELINES

NOTE: All per-serving nutritional information is based on one LEVEL I serving. LEVEL II and LEVEL III will vary, depending on portion size.

RECIPES

APRICOT SAUCE

1/2 cup apricot preserves
   1/8 cup Dijon mustard
     1/4 cup low-sodium soy sauce

Calories (kcal)	**56**
Total Fat	**‹1 g**
(3% calories from fat)	
Protein	**1 g**
Carbohydrate	**14 g**
Cholesterol	**0 mg**
Sodium	**353 mg**

Serves 8

In a small bowl, combine all ingredients and blend well.

LEVEL I
2 Tbsp. = 1 condiment

LEVEL II
3 Tbsp. = 1-1/2 condiments

LEVEL III
4 Tbsp. = 2 condiments

DIJONNAISE SAUCE

4 oz. nonfat yogurt
   4 oz. low-fat mayonnaise
     1 Tbsp. Dijon mustard
       1 tsp. chopped fresh dill
         2 tsp. Worcestershire sauce
           Black pepper (to taste)
             1 dash Tabasco® sauce

Calories (kcal)	**34**
Total Fat	**2 g**
(51% calories from fat)	
Protein	**1 g**
Carbohydrate	**3 g**
Cholesterol	**‹1 mg**
Sodium	**47 mg**

Serves 8

In a small bowl, combine all ingredients and blend well.

LEVEL I
2 Tbsp. = 1 condiment

LEVEL II
3 Tbsp. = 1-1/2 condiments

LEVEL III
4 Tbsp. = 2 condiments

MUSTARD CREAM SAUCE

per serving:

4 shallots, peeled and chopped
1-1/4 cups fat-free low-sodium chicken or vegetable broth
1-1/4 cups sweet vermouth
1/2 tsp. arrowroot powder
1/2 cup evaporated skim milk
1/4 cup Dijon mustard
1/2 tsp. salt
1 dash white pepper
1 Tbsp. chopped chives (for garnish)

Calories (kcal)..............**43**
Total Fat.....................**‹1 g**
(6% calories from fat)
Protein ....**2 g**
Carbohydrate ....**4 g**
Cholesterol ....**‹1 mg**
Sodium .... **164 mg**

Serves 8

1. Lightly coat the bottom of a saucepan with cooking spray and place over medium heat.

2. Add shallots and sauté until tender, using 1/4 cup of broth to deglaze pan as necessary.

3. Stir in remaining broth and vermouth. Simmer until reduced to 3/4 cup.

4. Dissolve arrowroot in a small amount of cold water and add to pan. Stir until slightly thickened.

5. Transfer sauce to a blender. Add evaporated milk, mustard, salt, and pepper and process until smooth. Garnish with chives.

LEVEL I	LEVEL II	LEVEL III
2 Tbsp. = 1 condiment	3 Tbsp. = 1-1/2 condiments	4 Tbsp. = 2 condiments

BARBECUE SAUCE

per serving:

1/4 cup ketchup
1/4 cup chili sauce
2 Tbsp. Worcestershire sauce
2 Tbsp. red wine vinegar
2 tsp. stone-ground mustard
1 tsp. dark brown sugar
1 dash cayenne pepper
2-1/2 tsp. crushed garlic

Calories (kcal)..............**16**
Total Fat.....................**‹1 g**
(1% calories from fat)
Protein ....**‹1 g**
Carbohydrate ....**4 g**
Cholesterol ....**0 mg**
Sodium .... **128 mg**

Serves 8

Whisk all ingredients together in a small bowl. Refrigerate until ready to use.

LEVEL I	LEVEL II	LEVEL III
2 Tbsp. = 1 condiment	3 Tbsp. = 1-1/2 condiments	4 Tbsp. = 2 condiments

BLUEBERRY MUFFINS

per serving:

1-3/4 cups whole wheat pastry flour
2-1/2 tsp. baking powder
1 cup powdered sugar
3/4 cup low-fat buttermilk
3 egg whites
1 cup thawed frozen blueberries (reserve juice)

Calories (kcal)............**167**	
Total Fat......................**1 g**	
(2% calories from fat)	
Protein ....**4 g**	
Carbohydrate ....**40 g**	
Cholesterol ....**1 mg**	
Sodium.................**135 mg**	

Serves 12

1. Preheat oven to 375° F. Line 12 muffin cups with paper liners.
2. In a small bowl, combine flour, baking powder, and sugar.
3. In a mixing bowl, whisk together buttermilk, egg whites, and 2 Tbsp. of reserved berry juice.
4. Add flour mixture to buttermilk mixture, stirring just to combine. Fold in berries.
5. Spoon batter into prepared muffin cups, mounding slightly. Bake until lightly browned, about 20 minutes.

LEVEL I	LEVEL II	LEVEL III
1 muffin = 1 carbohydrate	1 muffin = 1 carbohydrate	1 muffin = 1 carbohydrate

OATMEAL PANCAKES

per serving:

1/2 cup quick-cooking oats
1/2 cup low-fat buttermilk
1/2 cup skim milk
2 egg whites
1 Tbsp. canola oil
2 Tbsp. firmly packed brown sugar
Salt (to taste)
1 tsp. baking powder
1/2 cup whole wheat flour
1/2 cup all-purpose flour
1 tsp. cinnamon
1/2 tsp. baking soda

Calories (kcal)............**228**	
Total Fat......................**5 g**	
(19% calories from fat)	
Protein ....**9 g**	
Carbohydrate ....**37 g**	
Cholesterol ....**2 mg**	
Sodium.................**468 mg**	

Serves 4

1. In a medium bowl, combine oats, buttermilk, and milk. Set aside for 15 to 20 minutes to let oats absorb liquid.
2. In a separate bowl, beat together egg whites and oil. Add to oat mixture and mix together well. In small bowl, combine sugar, salt, cinnamon, baking powder, baking soda, and flour. Stir into oat mixture.
3. Heat a lightly oiled or nonstick griddle over medium-high heat (375 degrees for electric frying pan). Use 1/8 cup batter per pancake. Turn when tops bubble and edges look cooked. (Turn only once.)

LEVEL I	LEVEL II	LEVEL III
3 pancakes = 1 carbohydrate	3 pancakes = 1 carbohydrate	3 pancakes = 1 carbohydrate

BLACK AND WHITE BEAN CHILI

per serving:

1 tsp. canola oil

1 cup diced onion

2 cups fat-free low-sodium chicken or vegetable broth

6 oz. canned tomato paste

4 oz. green chilies, chopped

1 tsp. ground cumin

16 oz. canned black beans, rinsed and drained

16 oz. canned navy beans, rinsed and drained

Calories (kcal)............**202**

Total Fat.....................**2 g**

(8% calories from fat)

Protein ....**15 g**

Carbohydrate ....**35 g**

Cholesterol ....**0 mg**

Sodium.................**964 mg**

Serves 6

1. In a large soup pot, heat oil over medium-high heat. Add onions and cook for 5 minutes.

2. Add broth, tomato paste, chilies, cumin, and beans. Bring to a boil.

3. Reduce heat to low and simmer for 10 to 15 minutes, stirring occasionally.

LEVEL I
1 cup = 1 carbohydrate

LEVEL II
2 cups = 2 carbohydrates

LEVEL III
2 cups = 2 carbohydrates

GRILLED VEGGIE FOCACCIA

per serving:

1 large portobello mushroom, sliced thinly

1 large zucchini, sliced thinly

1 large yellow squash, sliced thinly

1-1/2 oz. part-skim mozzarella cheese, sliced

2 slices focaccia bread

Calories (kcal)............**284**

Total Fat.....................**9 g**

(28% calories from fat)

Protein ....**19 g**

Carbohydrate ....**33 g**

Cholesterol ....**23 mg**

Sodium.................**467 mg**

Serves 1

1. Grill or broil vegetables for 3 to 5 minutes using olive oil spray.

2. Place mozzarella cheese on one slice of bread, and toast under broiler or in toaster oven until cheese is melted.

3. Place vegetables on same side as cheese and top with second slice of bread. Serve.

LEVEL I
1 carbohydrate, 2 vegetables

LEVEL II
1 carbohydrate, 2 vegetables

LEVEL III
1 carbohydrate, 2 vegetables

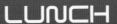

STUFFED BAKED POTATO

1 medium baking potato

10 oz. frozen chopped spinach

1/2 cup chopped broccoli

1 Tbsp. finely chopped green onions

1-1/2 oz. low-fat cheddar cheese

1 dash salt

1 dash pepper

1 dash garlic powder

Calories (kcal)............**167**	
Total Fat......................**1 g**	
(2% calories from fat)	
Protein ....**4 g**	
Carbohydrate ....**40 g**	
Cholesterol ....**1 mg**	
Sodium.................**135 mg**	

(Levels II & III, please double ingredients)

1. Bake potato at 425° F for 45 to 60 minutes, or microwave for about 8 minutes and then let stand for 3 to 5 minutes.
2. When potato is done, scoop its insides into a small bowl, reserving skin.
3. Add spinach, broccoli, green onions, cheese, and seasonings. Mash.
4. Fill potato skin with mixture and bake in oven 10 minutes longer to blend the flavors.

LEVEL I	LEVEL II	LEVEL III
1 potato = 1 carbohydrate, 1 vegetable, 1/2 dairy	2 potatoes = 2 carbohydrates, 2 vegetables, 1 dairy	2 potatoes = 2 carbohydrates, 2 vegetables, 1 dairy

PASTA SALAD—LEVEL I

2 oz. pasta

1 cup broccoli florets, steamed

2 whole green onions, chopped

1 Tbsp. olive oil

1 cup halved cherry tomatoes

1/2 tsp. fresh basil

1/4 tsp. garlic powder

1 oz. low-fat Parmesan cheese, grated

Calories (kcal)............**500**	
Total Fat....................**21 g**	
(32% calories from fat)	
Protein ....**17 g**	
Carbohydrate ....**65 g**	
Cholesterol ....**28 mg**	
Sodium.................**460 mg**	

1. Cook pasta according to directions on package. Drain.
2. While pasta cooks, steam broccoli.
3. In a bowl, combine cooked pasta, broccoli, green onions, olive oil, tomatoes, basil, and garlic powder. Mix well.
4. Sprinkle with cheese and toss again. Chill before serving.

LEVEL I	LEVEL II	LEVEL III
1 carbohydrate, 2 vegetables, 1 fat, 1/2 dairy	See next page	See next page

PASTA SALAD—LEVEL II

per serving:

3 oz. pasta
    1 cup broccoli florets, steamed
      2 whole green onions, chopped
        1-1/2 Tbsp. olive oil
          1 cup halved cherry tomatoes
            1/2 tsp. fresh basil
              1/4 tsp. garlic powder
                1 oz. low-fat Parmesan cheese, grated

Calories (kcal)	**666**
Total Fat	**28 g**
(43% calories from fat)	
Protein	**21 g**
Carbohydrate	**87 g**
Cholesterol	**28 mg**
Sodium	**462 mg**

1. Cook pasta according to directions on package. Drain.
2. While pasta cooks, steam broccoli.
3. In a bowl, combine cooked pasta, broccoli, green onions, olive oil, tomatoes, basil, and garlic powder. Mix well.
4. Sprinkle with cheese and toss again. Chill before serving.

LEVEL I
See previous page

LEVEL II
1-1/2 carbohydrates, 2 vegetables, 1-1/2 fats, 1/2 dairy

LEVEL III
See next below

PASTA SALAD—LEVEL III

per serving:

4 oz. pasta
    1-1/2 cup broccoli florets, steamed
      3 whole green onions, chopped
        2 Tbsp. olive oil
          1 cup halved cherry tomatoes
            1 tsp. fresh basil
              1/2 tsp. garlic powder
                1 oz. low-fat Parmesan cheese, grated

Calories (kcal)	**847**
Total Fat	**35 g**
(54% calories from fat)	
Protein	**26 g**
Carbohydrate	**111 g**
Cholesterol	**28 mg**
Sodium	**475 mg**

1. Cook pasta according to directions on package. Drain.
2. While pasta cooks, steam broccoli.
3. In bowl, combine cooked pasta, broccoli, green onions, olive oil, tomatoes, basil, and garlic powder. Mix well.
4. Sprinkle with cheese and toss again. Chill before serving.

LEVEL I
See previous page

LEVEL II
See above

LEVEL III
2 carbohydrates, 2 vegetables, 1-1/2 fats, 1/2 dairy

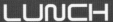

SPICY CHINESE NOODLES—LEVEL I

per serving:

2 oz. pasta
    2 Tbsp. chunky peanut butter
        1-1/2 Tbsp. low-sodium soy sauce
            1-1/2 Tbsp. rice vinegar
                1 tsp. honey
                    1 dash cayenne pepper
                        1 Tbsp. finely chopped green onions
                            Fat-free chicken broth (optional)

Calories (kcal)............**429**	
Total Fat....................**17 g**	
(35% calories from fat)	
Protein......................**16 g**	
Carbohydrate............**56 g**	
Cholesterol..............**0 mg**	
Sodium..............**1,056 mg**	

1. Cook pasta according to directions on package. Drain.
2. While pasta is cooking, combine peanut butter, soy sauce, vinegar, honey, and cayenne in a medium saucepan.
3. Add pasta to peanut butter sauce in pan and mix together. If pasta is too dry, add a little fat-free chicken broth to thin sauce. Garnish with green onions.

LEVEL I	LEVEL II	LEVEL III
1 protein, 1 carbohydrate, 1-1/2 fat	See below	See next page

SPICY CHINESE NOODLES—LEVEL II

per serving:

3 oz. pasta
    3 Tbsp. chunky peanut butter
        2 Tbsp. low-sodium soy sauce
            2 Tbsp. rice vinegar
                1-1/2 tsp. honey
                    1 dash cayenne pepper
                        2 Tbsp. finely chopped green onions
                            Fat-free chicken broth (optional)

Calories (kcal)............**660**	
Total Fat....................**26 g**	
(33% calories from fat)	
Protein......................**25 g**	
Carbohydrate............**89 g**	
Cholesterol..............**0 mg**	
Sodium..............**1,444 mg**	

1. Cook pasta according to directions on package. Drain.
2. While pasta is cooking, combine peanut butter, soy sauce, vinegar, honey, and cayenne in a medium saucepan.
3. Add pasta to peanut butter sauce in pan and mix together. If pasta is too dry, add a little fat-free chicken broth to thin sauce. Garnish with green onions.

LEVEL I	LEVEL II	LEVEL III
See above	1 protein, 1-1/2 carbohydrates, 2 fats	See next page

SPICY CHINESE NOODLES—LEVEL III

per serving:

4 oz. pasta

   3 Tbsp. chunky peanut butter

      3 Tbsp. low-sodium soy sauce

         3 Tbsp. rice vinegar

           2 tsp. honey

              1 dash cayenne pepper

                3 Tbsp. finely chopped green onions

                  Fat-free chicken broth (optional)

Calories (kcal)	**789**
Total Fat	**26 g**
(28% calories from fat)	
Protein	**29 g**
Carbohydrate	**115 g**
Cholesterol	**0 mg**
Sodium	**2,047 mg**

1. Cook pasta according to directions on package. Drain.
2. While pasta is cooking, combine peanut butter, soy sauce, vinegar, honey, and cayenne in a medium saucepan.
3. Add pasta to peanut butter sauce in pan and mix together. If pasta is too dry, add a little fat-free chicken broth to thin sauce. Garnish with green onions.

LEVEL I	LEVEL II	LEVEL III
See previous page	See previous page	1 protein, 2 carbohydrate, 2 fats

VEGETARIAN TOSTADA—LEVEL I

per serving:

1 large whole wheat tortilla

   1 cup fat-free canned refried beans

      1/4 cup diced tomato

         2 Tbsp. diced red onion

           1 cup shredded romaine lettuce

              2 Tbsp. low-fat sour cream

                2 Tbsp. salsa

Calories (kcal)	**449**
Total Fat	**7 g**
(14% calories from fat)	
Protein	**22 g**
Carbohydrate	**75 g**
Cholesterol	**6 mg**
Sodium	**1,437 mg**

1. Place large nonstick frying pan over medium heat.
2. Spray both sides of tortilla with corn oil spray and brown for several minutes on both sides until crisp.
3. Meanwhile, heat beans in a small saucepan.
4. Remove tortilla from pan. Place on plate and layer with beans, tomato, onion, lettuce, sour cream, and salsa. Serve.

LEVEL I	LEVEL II	LEVEL III
2 carbohydrates, 1 vegetable	See next page	See next page

PHASE 3—ENDURANCE MAXIMIZER

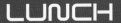

VEGETARIAN TOSTADA—LEVEL II

per serving:

1 large whole wheat tortilla
  1 cup fat-free canned refried beans
    1/2 cup cooked Spanish-style rice
      1/2 cup diced tomato
        3 Tbsp. diced red onion
          2 cups shredded romaine lettuce
            2 Tbsp. low-fat sour cream
              3 Tbsp. salsa

Calories (kcal)	**575**
Total Fat	**8 g**
(12% calories from fat)	
Protein	**25 g**
Carbohydrate	**102 g**
Cholesterol	**6 mg**
Sodium	**1,510 mg**

1. Place large nonstick frying pan over medium heat.
2. Spray both sides of tortilla with corn oil spray and brown for several minutes on both sides until crisp.
3. Meanwhile, heat beans in a small saucepan.
4. Remove tortilla from pan. Place on plate and layer with beans, rice, tomato, onion, lettuce, sour cream, and salsa. Serve.

LEVEL I	LEVEL II	LEVEL III
See previous page	2-1/2 carbohydrates, 2 vegetables	See below

VEGETARIAN TOSTADA—LEVEL III

per serving:

1 large whole wheat tortilla
  1 cup fat-free canned refried beans
    1 cup cooked Spanish-style rice
      1/2 cup diced tomato
        3 Tbsp. diced red onion
          2 cups shredded romaine lettuce
            2 Tbsp. low-fat sour cream
              3 Tbsp. salsa

Calories (kcal)	**701**
Total Fat	**8 g**
(10% calories from fat)	
Protein	**27 g**
Carbohydrate	**130 g**
Cholesterol	**6 mg**
Sodium	**1,510 mg**

1. Place large nonstick frying pan over medium heat.
2. Spray both sides of tortilla with corn oil spray and brown for several minutes on both sides until crisp.
3. Meanwhile, heat beans in a small saucepan.
4. Remove tortilla from pan. Place on plate and layer with beans, rice, tomato, onion, lettuce, sour cream, and salsa. Serve.

LEVEL I	LEVEL II	LEVEL III
See previous page	See above	3 carbohydrates, 2 vegetables

MEDITERRANEAN SHRIMP KEBABS—LEVEL I

per serving:

6 shrimp (1 ounce each)

1/8 red onion, cubed

1/2 zucchini, cut in 1-inch-thick slices

1/4 yellow pepper, seeded and diced

4 white button mushrooms

1/4 cup fresh lemon juice

1 Tbsp. olive oil

1 tsp. oregano

2 metal or wooden skewers

Calories (kcal)............**349**

Total Fat....................**17 g**

(42% calories from fat)

Protein ....**36 g**

Carbohydrate ....**14 g**

Cholesterol ....**259 mg**

Sodium................**257 mg**

1. Assemble kebabs by alternating vegetables and shrimp, using three shrimp per skewer.
2. In a small bowl, blend lemon juice, olive oil, and oregano to make a marinade.
3. Brush marinade over kebabs; place kebabs on grill for 7 to 10 minutes.
4. Turn and brush with remaining marinade while grilling until vegetables are cooked
   and shrimp are opaque.

LEVEL I	LEVEL II	LEVEL III
2 protein, 1 vegetable, 1 fat	See below	See next page

MEDITERRANEAN SHRIMP KEBABS—LEVEL II

per serving:

9 shrimp (1 ounce each)

1/8 red onion, cubed

1/2 zucchini, cut in 1-inch-thick slices

1/4 yellow pepper, seeded and diced

6 white button mushrooms

1/4 cup fresh lemon juice

1 Tbsp. olive oil

1 tsp. oregano

3 metal or wooden skewers

Calories (kcal)............**449**

Total Fat....................**7 g**

(14% calories from fat)

Protein ....**22 g**

Carbohydrate ....**75 g**

Cholesterol ....**6 mg**

Sodium..............**1,437 mg**

1. Assemble kebabs by alternating vegetables and shrimp, using three shrimp per skewer.
2. In a small bowl, blend lemon juice, olive oil, and oregano to make a marinade.
3. Brush marinade over kebabs; place kebabs on grill for 7 to 10 minutes.
4. Turn and brush with remaining marinade while grilling until vegetables are cooked
   and shrimp are opaque.

LEVEL I	LEVEL II	LEVEL III
See above	3 protein, 1 vegetable, 1 fat	See next page

PHASE 3—ENDURANCE MAXIMIZER

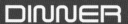

MEDITERRANEAN SHRIMP KEBABS—LEVEL III

per serving:

12 shrimp (1 ounce each)
1/8 red onion, cubed
1/2 zucchini, cut in 1-inch-thick slices
1/4 yellow pepper, seeded and diced
8 white button mushrooms
1/4 cup fresh lemon juice
1 Tbsp. olive oil
1 tsp. oregano
4 metal or wooden skewers

Calories (kcal)	**636**
Total Fat	**27 g**
(1% calories from fat)	
Protein	**73 g**
Carbohydrate	**28 g**
Cholesterol	**517 mg**
Sodium	**513 mg**

1. Assemble kebabs by alternating vegetables and shrimp, using three shrimp per skewer.
2. In a small bowl, blend lemon juice, olive oil, and oregano to make a marinade.
3. Brush marinade over kebabs; place kebabs on grill for 7 to 10 minutes.
4. Turn and brush with remaining marinade while grilling until vegetables are cooked
   and shrimp are opaque.

LEVEL I	LEVEL II	LEVEL III
See previous page	See previous page	4 protein, 1 vegetable, 1 fat

PORK CHOP BAKED WITH APPLE AND SWEET POTATO—LEVEL I

per serving:

6 oz. lean boneless pork loin
1 medium sweet potato
1 medium apple
Pinch cinnamon (optional)
Pinch salt (optional)
Pinch black pepper (optional)

Calories (kcal)	**415**
Total Fat	**8 g**
(17% calories from fat)	
Protein	**33 g**
Carbohydrate	**53 g**
Cholesterol	**77 mg**
Sodium	**80 mg**

1. Preheat oven to 350° F.
2. Slice sweet potato thinly. Core apple and slice it into eight pieces.
3. On a large piece of foil, layer sweet potato slices, pork chop, then apple slices.
   If desired, sprinkle with cinnamon, salt, and pepper.
4. Wrap well and bake for 40 minutes.

LEVEL I	LEVEL II	LEVEL III
2 protein, 1 carbohydrate, 1 fruit	See next page	See next page

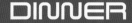

PORK CHOP BAKED WITH APPLE AND SWEET POTATO—LEVEL II

per serving:

9 oz. lean boneless pork loin
    1 medium sweet potato
        1 medium apple
            Pinch cinnamon (optional)
                Pinch salt (optional)
                    Pinch black pepper (optional)

Calories (kcal)	**513**
Total Fat	**12 g**
(21% calories from fat)	
Protein	**48 g**
Carbohydrate	**53 g**
Cholesterol	**115 mg**
Sodium	**111 mg**

1. Preheat oven to 350° F.
2. Slice sweet potato thinly. Core apple and slice it into eight pieces.
3. On a large piece of foil, layer sweet potato slices, pork chop, then apple slices.
   If desired, sprinkle with cinnamon, salt, and pepper.
4. Wrap well and bake for 40 minutes.

LEVEL I	LEVEL II	LEVEL III
See previous page	2 protein, 1 carbohydrate, 1 fruit	See below

PORK CHOP BAKED WITH APPLE AND SWEET POTATO—LEVEL III

per serving:

12 oz. lean boneless pork loin
    1 medium sweet potato
        1 medium apple
            Pinch cinnamon (optional)
                Pinch salt (optional)
                    Pinch black pepper (optional)

Calories (kcal)	**611**
Total Fat	**16 g**
(23% calories from fat)	
Protein	**63 g**
Carbohydrate	**53 g**
Cholesterol	**153 mg**
Sodium	**142 mg**

1. Preheat oven to 350° F.
2. Slice sweet potato thinly. Core apple and slice it into eight pieces.
3. On a large piece of foil, layer sweet potato slices, pork chop, then apple slices.
   If desired, sprinkle with cinnamon, salt, and pepper.
4. Wrap well and bake for 40 minutes.

LEVEL I	LEVEL II	LEVEL III
See previous page	See above	4 protein, 1 carbohydrate, 1 fruit

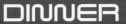

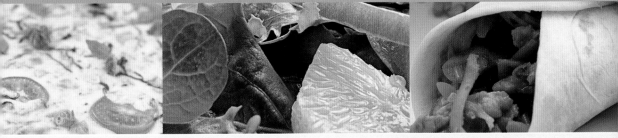

QUICK OPTIONS

CONVENIENCE FOODS
GUIDELINES

If you just don't have the time to prepare anything more elaborate than toast, here are some brands you can consider the next time you hit the frozen food section. These foods can be used sparingly when needed, but do not exceed more than one per day.

_Amy's Kitchen®
_Weight Watchers® Smart Ones®
_Lean Cuisine®
_Cascadian Farm®
_Cedarlane® Natural Food
_Healthy Choice®

Follow the calorie, fat, and sodium guidelines below:

LEVEL I	1,800 CALORIES	Up to 400 calories per meal	10 g fat	600 mg sodium
LEVEL II	2,400 CALORIES	Up to 600 calories per meal	12 g fat	800 mg sodium
LEVEL III	3,000 CALORIES	Up to 800 calories per meal	15 g fat	1,000 mg sodium

Amy's Kitchen, Weight Watchers, Smart Ones, Lean Cuisine, Cascadian Farm, Cedarlane, and Healthy Choice are registered trademarks of their respective owners.

QUICK AT-HOME DISHES

Try these quick, healthy, and tasty dishes that are a snap to prepare.

		SERVING SIZE	
SOFT TACOS	Chicken Corn tortillas Salsa	6 oz. 2 to taste	2 protein 1 carbohydrate 1 condiment
STIR-FRY	Shrimp or chicken Rice Vegetables Soy sauce	6 oz. 1 cup 1 cup to taste	2 protein 1 carbohydrate 1 vegetable 1 condiment
TUNA SALAD	Tuna Bread Salad greens Fat-free dressing or mayo	6 oz. 2 slices 2 cups 2 Tbsp.	2 protein 1 carbohydrate 1 vegetable 1 condiment
BURGER	Soy or turkey burger Lettuce, tomato, onion Ketchup and mustard	1 to taste to taste	2 protein 1 vegetable 1 condiment

QUICK OPTIONS

CALORIE AND GRAM BREAKDOWN

The P90X Nutrition Plan is designed to work without having to worry about a lot of math. The portion plans keep fiber, vitamins, and minerals high, while keeping cholesterol, sodium, and bad fats low. But if you're someone who likes to be a little more DIY with your nutrition, this is the information you'll need.

If you're going to build a diet yourself based purely on these numbers, you really need to know what you're doing. If you know how to do that, go for it. If not, we recommend using our plans as a base.

CALORIES

			PROTEIN	CARBS	FAT
PHASE 1 FAT SHREDDER	LEVEL I	1,800 calories	900 calories	540 calories	360 calories
	LEVEL II	2,400 calories	1,200 calories	720 calories	480 calories
	LEVEL III	3,000 calories	1,500 calories	900 calories	600 calories
PHASE 2 ENERGY BOOSTER	LEVEL I	1,800 calories	720 calories	720 calories	360 calories
	LEVEL II	2,400 calories	960 calories	960 calories	480 calories
	LEVEL III	3,000 calories	1,200 calories	1,200 calories	600 calories
PHASE 3 ENDURANCE MAXIMIZER	LEVEL I	1,800 calories	360 calories	1,080 calories	360 calories
	LEVEL II	2,400 calories	480 calories	1,440 calories	480 calories
	LEVEL III	3,000 calories	600 calories	1,800 calories	600 calories

To convert those calories into grams, we used the following equations:

1 gram of protein = 4 calories • 1 gram of carbohydrates = 4 calories • 1 gram of fat = 9 calories

Keep in mind, your body isn't a computer. It doesn't need, nor understand, exact numbers—if your daily carb, protein, and fat grams aren't on the nose, it doesn't matter. In other words, whether you're counting percentages, calories, or grams, just get in the ballpark with your macronutrients and you'll be fine. In fact, varying nutrients can avoid potential plateaus. Also, keeping a daily log will help you figure out the best ways to fine-tune your eating.

GRAMS

			PROTEIN	CARBS	FAT
PHASE1 FAT SHREDDER	LEVEL I	1,800 calories	225 g	135 g	40 g
	LEVEL II	2,400 calories	300 g	180 g	53 g
	LEVEL III	3,000 calories	375 g	225 g	67 g
PHASE2 ENERGY BOOSTER	LEVEL I	1,800 calories	180 g	180 g	40 g
	LEVEL II	2,400 calories	240 g	240 g	53 g
	LEVEL III	3,000 calories	300 g	300 g	67 g
PHASE3 ENDURANCE MAXIMIZER	LEVEL I	1,800 calories	90 g	270 g	40 g
	LEVEL II	2,400 calories	120 g	360 g	53 g
	LEVEL III	3,000 calories	150 g	450 g	67 g

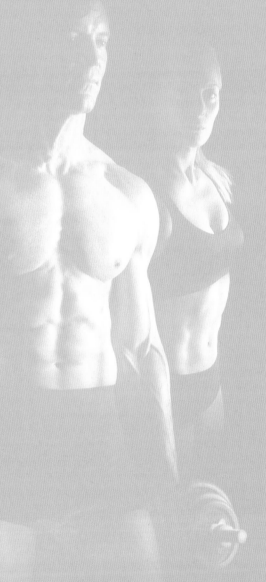

Staying true to the eating approach you've selected for this plan is more important to your P90X success than anything else. Deviating from the healthy, targeted nutrition plan outlined for you is NOT an option. One of the best ways to keep on track and stay within the parameters of your nutrition level is to maintain a daily journal. What and how much you choose to write is up to you. Just be sure to indicate how successful you were for each specific day.

DAILY JOURNAL

BREAKFAST	SNACK	LUNCH	SNACK	DINNER	COMMENTS	
						_MO
						_TU
						_WE
						_TH
						_FR
						_SA
						_SU

BREAKFAST	SNACK	LUNCH	SNACK	DINNER	COMMENTS	
						_MO
						_TU
						_WE
						_TH
						_FR
						_SA
						_SU

	BREAKFAST	SNACK	LUNCH	SNACK	DINNER	COMMENTS
_MO						
_TU						
_WE						
_TH						
_FR						
_SA						
_SU						

	BREAKFAST	SNACK	LUNCH	SNACK	DINNER	COMMENTS
_MO						
_TU						
_WE						
_TH						
_FR						
_SA						
_SU						

BREAKFAST	SNACK	LUNCH	SNACK	DINNER	COMMENTS	
						_MO
						_TU
						_WE
						_TH
						_FR
						_SA
						_SU

BREAKFAST	SNACK	LUNCH	SNACK	DINNER	COMMENTS	
						_MO
						_TU
						_WE
						_TH
						_FR
						_SA
						_SU

	BREAKFAST	SNACK	LUNCH	SNACK	DINNER	COMMENTS
_MO						
_TU						
_WE						
_TH						
_FR						
_SA						
_SU						

	BREAKFAST	SNACK	LUNCH	SNACK	DINNER	COMMENTS
_MO						
_TU						
_WE						
_TH						
_FR						
_SA						
_SU						

BREAKFAST	SNACK	LUNCH	SNACK	DINNER	COMMENTS	
						_MO
						_TU
						_WE
						_TH
						_FR
						_SA
						_SU

BREAKFAST	SNACK	LUNCH	SNACK	DINNER	COMMENTS	
						_MO
						_TU
						_WE
						_TH
						_FR
						_SA
						_SU

	BREAKFAST	SNACK	LUNCH	SNACK	DINNER	COMMENTS
_MO						
_TU						
_WE						
_TH						
_FR						
_SA						
_SU						

	BREAKFAST	SNACK	LUNCH	SNACK	DINNER	COMMENTS
_MO						
_TU						
_WE						
_TH						
_FR						
_SA						
_SU						

BREAKFAST	SNACK	LUNCH	SNACK	DINNER	COMMENTS	
						_MO
						_TU
						_WE
						_TH
						_FR
						_SA
						_SU

BREAKFAST	SNACK	LUNCH	SNACK	DINNER	COMMENTS	
						_MO
						_TU
						_WE
						_TH
						_FR
						_SA
						_SU

	BREAKFAST	SNACK	LUNCH	SNACK	DINNER	COMMENTS
_MO						
_TU						
_WE						
_TH						
_FR						
_SA						
_SU						

	BREAKFAST	SNACK	LUNCH	SNACK	DINNER	COMMENTS
_MO						
_TU						
_WE						
_TH						
_FR						
_SA						
_SU						

RECIPE INDEX